Lessons Learned for Provisioning and Delivering U.S. Military Behavioral Health Care, 2003–2013

KRISTIE L. GORE, RYAN ANDREW BROWN, KATHRYN O'CONNOR

Prepared for the Center for Deployment Psychology at the Uniformed
Services University of the Health Sciences
Approved for public release; distribution unlimited

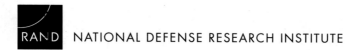

RAND NATIONAL DEFENSE RESEARCH INSTITUTE

For more information on this publication, visit www.rand.org/t/RRA391-1

Library of Congress Cataloging-in-Publication Data is available for this publication.
ISBN: 978-1-9774-0651-4

Published by the RAND Corporation, Santa Monica, Calif.
© Copyright 2021 RAND Corporation
RAND® is a registered trademark.

Cover: U.S. Army.

Support RAND
Make a tax-deductible charitable contribution at
www.rand.org/giving/contribute

www.rand.org

Preface

The behavioral health demands stemming from the longstanding wars in Iraq and Afghanistan led to significant changes in the provision and delivery of behavioral health care in the U.S. military. The Center for Deployment Psychology (CDP) at the Uniformed Services University of the Health Sciences (USUHS) commissioned the RAND Corporation to conduct interviews with experts to capture lessons learned that could help prepare future military behavioral health providers. RAND reviewed publicly available material to identify events and circumstances that prompted those changes. That material informed the selection of interviewees. This report highlights select events and insights of experts regarding the lessons they learned between 2003 and 2013 about the provision and delivery of military behavioral health care.

The research reported here was completed in July 2020 and underwent security review with the sponsor and the Defense Office of Prepublication and Security Review before public release.

This research was sponsored by the USUHS CDP and conducted within the Forces and Resources Policy Center of the RAND National Security Research Division (NSRD), which operates the National Defense Research Institute (NDRI), a federally funded research and development center sponsored by the Office of the Secretary of Defense, the Joint Staff, the Unified Combatant Commands, the Navy, the Marine Corps, the defense agencies, and the defense intelligence enterprise.

For more information on the RAND Forces and Resources Policy Center, see www.rand.org/nsrd/frp or contact the director (contact information is provided on the webpage).

Contents

Summary

Background

The Center for Deployment Psychology (CDP) at the Uniformed Services University of the Health Sciences sponsored this effort to conduct interviews with experts to capture lessons learned that could help prepare future military behavioral health providers. We aimed to collect the lessons that U.S. Department of Defense (DoD) health care providers and administrators of behavioral health care had learned during the first ten years of U.S. military campaigns in Afghanistan and Iraq. Our goal was to establish the groundwork for future investigation into the major events, policy shifts, and effects on practice.

Approach

We first reviewed policies, reports, academic literature, and media sources to identify significant events in military behavioral health between 2003 and 2013 (i.e., during operations Enduring Freedom, Iraqi Freedom, and New Dawn). We developed structured procedures for identifying and describing key events associated with the provision and delivery of military behavioral health care. We identified events from the background material and sorted them into the following categories: media events, policies, government and academic reports, ethics of operational psychology, organizational changes, and resources, for a total of 96 events. Seven were journal articles.

Through that work, we identified significant developments in military behavioral health care, selected 42 experts who could address these developments, and interviewed 17 of them. Our interviewees provided a rich descriptive history of their experiences related to military behavioral health care. The interviewees detailed many of the areas in which change occurred and identified lessons that could help prepare the U.S. military behavioral health workforce for future conflicts. These individuals had long military careers, spanning many roles. If we had attempted to capture the totality of the lessons they had learned, interviews could have occurred over multiple days.

Limitations and Scope

Expert input is inherently subjective. The interviewees conveyed their own opinions, and we drew inferences from their experiences. Because of time, budget, and regulatory constraints, we did not rely on a structured qualitative analysis. Nonetheless, we provide here a selection of lessons learned that lend themselves to initial insights based on a limited set of interviews and events.

Interviewee Insights on Provisioning Military Behavioral Health Care

During the 2003–2013 period, manpower shortfalls made it difficult to meet the demand for behavioral health services—with problems stemming both from the inability to estimate requirements and difficulty accessing providers. Interviewees discussed obstacles and solutions for building a provider pipeline (using scholarships, retention bonuses, and other financial incentives) and for hiring the needed number and mix of providers. The overall lesson interviewees described seems to be that it is possible to surge to meet new demands on the behavioral health system, but doing so requires avenues for hiring and appropriate incentives. The interviewees described several lessons about the provision of behavioral health care between 2003 and 2013:

- Tools to predict manpower requirements were needed.
- It is important to properly incentivize professional psychologist involvement in military careers and to engage human resources early and often in psychologists' career development so that they are aware of and attracted to military careers.
- DoD requires direct hire authority for behavioral health care specialists to support major overseas contingency operations.
- Psychologists must be licensed before deploying.
- A single coordinating authority is needed that can prescribe what training and education behavioral health providers should get and the modality (institutional training, mobile training, continuing education) by which they should get it.
- Operational psychologists need clear guidance on adherence to ethical practices within their operational support roles.
- Embedded behavioral health care is critical for establishing rapport, early intervention, and effective care.
- Providers need to be prepared to operate as organic assets, assigned to a unit, and to communicate their value and role to commanders and service members.
- Providers need to know the contents of and how to use the latest clinical practice guidelines and assessment instruments as these tools continue to evolve.
- Efforts to streamline and reduce the time required for regulatory review of behavioral health studies could bring health solutions to service members sooner.

Interviewee Insights on Delivering Military Behavioral Health Care

From their own experience, the interviewees offered several lessons about the delivery of military behavioral health care:

- Behavioral health providers need to be prepared to practice in military treatment facilities, in theater, and in different roles, depending on the setting (i.e., primary care, specialty care, and consultation).

- A center of excellence for behavioral health needs to be empowered to coordinate services within the Military Health System.
- Behavioral health providers need to be prepared to address prevention and health within a nonmedical model.
- Integration of behavioral and nonbehavioral health care is critical.
- Behavioral health providers need to be prepared to practice in the primary-care setting.
- It is important for military behavioral health providers to be effective assessment technicians during all touch points and to feel competent delivering preclinical interventions to build resilience among the military population.
- Behavioral health providers need to be able to articulate their role and value to commanders, understand confidentiality policies, and communicate the minimum necessary information to address the information commanders need to know to maintain unit readiness.
- Behavioral health providers need to be trained to follow Department of Veterans Affairs and DoD clinical practice guidelines for the treatment of posttraumatic stress disorder, depression, and other psychological disorders in service members and their families.
- Behavioral health providers need to be prepared to document care delivery using standardized tools conducive to measuring the quality of their care.
- Families need support through multiple and frequent deployment cycles.

Conclusion

These results can help guide how CDP and DoD prepare future behavioral health providers to care for future warriors and their families. The findings stemming from this effort to understand lessons from the complex and fluid events surrounding the delivery of behavioral health care during 2003–2013 can be viewed as research questions in need of evaluation. We selected the events that seemed most influential, the interviewees, the interview topics (with CDP), and interview excerpts from a wealth of material the experts provided. Subsequent researchers repeating this process would likely derive different takeaways from another group of events and experts.

Despite efforts to trace major changes and drivers of those changes, we undoubtedly did not identify other significant events. There is more to be learned from the individuals we interviewed, and we are missing many important perspectives and lessons from those we did not interview. We hope that future work may build on our data and analysis. Interviewees also discussed topics other than the provision and delivery of military behavioral health care; for instance, several interviewees described the importance of standardized program implementation procedures. We excluded such topics when selecting interview excerpts. It is also important to empirically evaluate the lessons described here. Further research on the effectiveness of policy and practice responses to evolving behavioral health demands is warranted. Research on the effectiveness of embedded care delivery models, training programs, and quality of care may validate the opinions of the experts we interviewed. Some interviewees pointed out that better anticipating events, to be proactive instead of reactive, is critical going forward. As Dr. Eric Getka put it, "looking back is extremely valuable, but trying to look forward to anticipate what the psychological needs of the future warfighter are going to be is just as important."[1]

---

[1]   Interview with Dr. Eric Getka, February 11, 2020.

Acknowledgments

This work was made possible by the sponsorship and support of the Executive Director of the Center for Deployment Psychology (CDP), David Riggs. We are grateful for his support and for the support of our project monitor, Director of CDP, William Brim. We wish to thank the many experts who provided indispensable input during formulation of the research and on the events and data sources: In addition to our interviewees, these were Lisa French, Jenna Ermold, COL Christopher Ivany, and Charles Engel. This project benefited from RAND Quality Assurance reviews by Lisa Harrington, Molly McIntosh, John Winkler, Craig Bond, and James Powers and from peer reviews by Matthew Wade Markel of RAND and Carl Castro of the University of Southern California.

We want to express our gratitude to the following experts, who took the time to share their extensive experiences and insights with us:

- Peter Chiarelli
- David Chu
- Bruce Crow
- Michael Dinneen
- Charles Engel
- Eric Getka
- Carroll Greene
- David Kieran
- Robert Lippy
- William Nash
- David Orman
- Mark Paris
- Rebecca Porter
- David Riggs
- Eric Schoomaker
- Terri Tanielian
- Jonathan Woodson

They generously shared their ideas about the delivery of behavioral health care during the wars in Iraq and Afghanistan. Their tremendous contributions to military medicine are reflected in their biographies, which appear in Appendix D.

It is our hope that documenting their experiences will enable future generations to respond to the behavioral health demands of war by implementing the lessons of the past instead of having to relearn them.

CHAPTER ONE

Introduction

Background

It is instructive for the U.S. military to take stock of what has been learned about providing military behavioral health care during wartime. In the face of long and repeated combat deployments, U.S. service members and their families withstood incredible stressors, which increased the demand for behavioral health services. This report aims to capture some of the lessons learned from a review of publicly available material related to changes in the delivery of military behavioral health care between 2003 and 2013 and from interviews with experts and front-line practitioners involved in these changes.

The military behavioral health system necessarily evolved to meet the demands of the high operational tempo (OPTEMPO) and the extensive "invisible wounds" of combat deployers (Tanielian and Jaycox, 2008). It is important to understand why the health system evolved; how it evolved; whether (and how) that evolution was valuable; and, in hindsight, what decisions could (or should) have been different. Many lessons about caring for the psychological and emotional needs of warriors and their families, barriers to care, and techniques to overcome these barriers can be captured by identifying the drivers of change and hearing from the individuals who lived through the changes. As large-scale combat deployments are reduced and as the deployment of behavioral health care assets is changing, there is a risk that these lessons could be lost to history if not documented.

The Center for Deployment Psychology (CDP) interacts with thousands of military and civilian providers annually who provide behavioral health care to warriors, veterans, and their families. Created in 2006 to ensure a prepared behavioral health workforce, the CDP's mission is to lead the development of a community of culturally mindful and clinically competent providers through the delivery of high-quality training and education, the convening of experts, and the dissemination of research-based treatment and the latest topics in military behavioral health. CDP accomplishes this through the development and dissemination of resources and training materials and through consultation and outreach to health care providers. In part through this project, CDP now aims to capture key reflections from U.S. Department of Defense (DoD) behavioral health care providers, trainers, administrators, and policymakers who served during operations Iraqi Freedom (OIF) and Enduring Freedom (OEF) between 2003 and 2013.

As CDP looks toward meeting the educational and training needs to prepare behavioral health providers, it is important to reflect on what was learned regarding the provisioning, equipping, training, delivering of behavioral health care both in theatre and in garrison between 2003 and 2013. Asking these questions of DoD health care providers who had administered behavioral health care during OIF and OEF provides an opportunity to retain these lessons and experiences.

Behavioral health care delivery in OIF and OEF followed a fast-paced, complex, and fluid path. Many events occurred behind the scenes, including changes in leadership, military strategy, care delivery models, and health system organization. It is challenging to distill lessons in the face of so much evolution and turmoil. In April 2019, Dr. David Kieran published a seminal book, *Signature Wounds: The Untold Story of the Military's Mental Health Crisis* (Kieran, 2019). This 404-page book is a detailed depiction of the events that occurred during the period we cover in this report. Kieran collected thousands of references, pursued Freedom of Information Act requests, and conducted roughly 50 interviews with key individuals to describe the events and experiences surrounding military behavioral health care. Although the book does not specifically address the experiences of behavioral health providers, it describes important events and senior leader opinions in detail and over a longer time frame than we do here. It is an important resource and an example of the importance of documenting this history. When we interviewed Kieran,[1] he told us the book took him five years to complete, including a one-year full-time fellowship. We refer the interested reader to the book for further background on the U.S. military's experiences with behavioral health.

There are and will be many accounts of lessons learned from the longest wars the United States has seen. Given the focus on service members' behavioral health and readiness, there is much to be gleaned from changes and progress during OIF and OEF. For instance, Reger and Moore, 2006, reported on four lessons they had learned using combat stress control (CSC) in Iraq:

1. Commanders' need for personnel strength may reduce likelihood of consulting with behavioral health providers. Thus, "selling" the utility of CSC as a force multiplier may be necessary.
2. Placement of CSC personnel should be flexible and able to adapt to changing battlefield conditions.
3. Regular needs assessments can help CSC anticipate problems from changing conditions.
4. It is important to make people (commanders and providers) aware of CSC services.

Reger and Moore also offered recommendations, such as predeployment training for psychologists in preparing a case disposition rationale for commanders, as well as marketing ideas for communicating the presence and capabilities of CSC (Reger and Moore, 2006).

Objective

We interviewed and collected the lessons that DoD health care providers and administrators of behavioral health care had learned from the first ten years of the U.S. military campaigns in Afghanistan and Iraq. Our goal is for these lessons to contribute to further evaluation

---

[1] Interview with Dr. David Kieran, April 10, 2020.

and the preparation of behavioral health providers for future wartime situations. We relied on a literature review and expert consultation to select interviewees who could offer important lessons regarding providing and delivering behavioral health services. The goal was to organize and describe the interviewees' insights as they pertain to preparing the future behavioral health workforce.

Approach

To focus our interviews, we first reviewed policies, reports, the academic literature, and media sources to identify significant events in military behavioral health between 2003 and 2013 (during OEF and OIF). We developed structured procedures for identifying and describing key events associated with the provision and delivery of military behavioral health care. We standardized our background material data-collection procedures so that others could follow them in the future. We developed two conceptual frameworks: one to organize the background material we identified (sorting them into the categories of media, policies, government and academic reports, ethics of operational psychology, organizational changes, and resources) and another to organize the insights from the interviewees (provision topics and care delivery topics). We collected 96 events, of which 27 were policies; 17 were about ethics in operational psychology; 15 were reports; 14 were resources; ten were organizational changes; seven were journal articles, and six were media events. At the request of the sponsor, CDP, we developed two databases: One is a timeline of key events in the delivery of behavioral health care based on background material we identified, and one is a collection of interviews (and transcripts) that can be used in perpetuity to derive lessons the interviewees learned.[2]

We also consulted experts to find materials we missed. Through that work, we identified significant developments and shifts in military behavioral health care. These drove the selection of 42 experts who could address the developments, and we conducted interviews with 17

---

[2]   Methods for developing the timeline are available on request.

of these experts. Our interviewees described their experiences related to military behavioral health care; detailed many of the areas in which change occurred; and areas identified lessons that would help prepare the U.S. military behavioral health workforce for future wars. The interviews lasted approximately 90 minutes.

The interviewees had long careers in or working with the military, spanning many roles. If we attempted to capture the totality of the lessons they learned, interviews could have occurred over multiple days. We discussed potential topic areas with interviewees prior to taping to derive specific topics they deemed most important and we deemed most relevant for our purposes. Appendix D provides biographies for the individuals we interviewed. Each has a distinguished career spanning a combined total of about one thousand years of military health care delivery, operations, and policy experience.

Scope

We necessarily limited the time frame and the depth with which we could examine different aspects of this broad and complex topic. The significant events and policies were limited to the provision and delivery of behavioral health care. To establish some boundaries for this effort, we selected the period beginning with the 2003 invasion of Iraq and ending about 2013, during the force drawdown in Afghanistan. Undoubtedly, this time frame meant missing some important lessons. We excluded specific topics that are not as central to the delivery of military behavioral health care, such as TRICARE practices and reimbursement rates and the epidemiology of psychological problems in service members.

Limitations

Expert input is inherently subjective. The interviewees conveyed their opinions and experiences, from which we drew inferences. Because of time, budget, and regulatory constraints, we did not rely on a structured qualitative analysis. A qualitative interview study that relied on a standardized protocol for thematic and content analysis would have required survey licensing and a larger budget. The sponsor preferred to capture unique opinions, as in an oral history. This report provides a sampling of lessons learned that lends itself to initial insights based on a limited set of interviews and events. There are undoubtedly other significant events that we did not identify, despite efforts to trace major changes and their drivers. There is more to be learned from the individuals we interviewed. The lessons we have derived from the interviews are also subjective. The portions of interviews described in this report reflect our own views on what is important and actionable. We are missing many important perspectives and lessons from those we did not interview. We hope that future work may build on our data and analysis.

Organization of this Report

The remainder of this report presents the results of our work. In Chapter Two, we describe the major events and shifts in military behavioral health care that we identified in background review. We report on interviewees' insights about provisioning care in Chapter Three and in delivering care in Chapter Four. In Chapter Five, we reflect on the background material and the interviews, describe where behavioral health care began in 2003 and how it has evolved, and conclude with a call for future efforts to build on this work. We include the interview procedures, protocol, and release form in Appendixes A, B, and C, respectively. Appendix D contains biographies of all the interviewees.

CHAPTER TWO

Contextual Events

This chapter describes some of the significant events and shifts in the delivery of behavioral health care between 2003 and 2013 that we identified in our review of publicly available sources. We describe some of the major events and developments in the categories we established for such events. Most of these events led us to identify experts that could discuss the topics in detail.

Media

Media attention begets leadership attention, and high-profile tragedies are met with public scrutiny and the need for a public military response. One high-profile incident that demanded a response from military leadership was the abuse of detainees at Abu Ghraib in September 2004. The story prompted concern about service member behavioral health and behavior; it also introduced the military's handling of detainees to the general public. What followed was growing attention on the ethics of operational psychology (discussed later) and the tensions between the American Psychological Association (APA) and the U.S. military regarding the roles that psychologists may ethically play.

Among the other high-profile events were many public tragedies, including a string of homicides at Fort Carson, Colorado, which led to an important investigative review by a multidisciplinary team from the U.S. Army Public Health Command. Between 2005 and 2008, 14 soldiers from Fort Carson were convicted of 11 homicides and two attempted murders. In 2009, the epidemiologic consulting (EPICON) was conducted to investigate the murders (U.S. Army Center for Health Promotion and Preventive Medicine, 2009). The investigative team had aimed to discover any correlation and causation between deployment overseas and the violent outbreaks. Of the 14 soldiers, ten had been diagnosed with behavioral health conditions prior to the homicides. Among other findings, the team reported that "a combination of individual, unit, and environmental factors converged to increase the population risk in the index BCT [brigade combat team] which made clustering of negative outcomes more likely" (U.S. Army Center for Health Promotion and Preventive Medicine, 2009, p. ES-4).

In February 2007, the *Washington Post* reported on the poor living conditions at Walter Reed Army Medical Center, where service members were being treated for war-related injuries and going through disability evaluation processes. DoD's response included building reforms and changes in the management of the disability evaluation system. For example, medical hold and medical holdover became the Warrior Transition Brigade (President's Commission on Care for America's Returning Wounded Warriors, 2007).

Policies

A string of murder-suicides at Fort Bragg, North Carolina, in summer 2002 heightened sensitivities around the mental health consequences of combat. The investigations of these events precipitated the first mental health advisor team (MHAT) and the introduction of behavioral health screening questions in 2003 on the Post Deployment Health Assessment (DD 2796). Pre- and postdeployment health assessments and reassessments evolved to improve the monitoring of behavioral health before and after deployment. Section 735 of the fiscal year (FY) 2007 National Defense Authorization Act (NDAA) (Pub. L. 109-364, 2006) required behavioral health assessments to include the specific behavioral health needs of those deployed in OIF or OEF on their return. This included identifying behavioral health conditions (posttraumatic stress disorder [PTSD], suicide) among those who served multiple deployments, evaluation of the availability of assessments to detect behavioral health conditions that may emerge over time, and recommendations for improving behavioral health services for affected service members. Section 708 in the FY 2010 NDAA (Pub. L. 111-84, 2009) first required the use of the a person-to-person review of the DD 2796 Post-Deployment Mental Health Assessment and included policies for how the assessment should be administered and shared between the DoD and the Department of Veterans Affairs (VA). The Assistant Secretary of Defense for Health Affairs provided further clarification in 2010 and 2011 through a series of memorandums, before the Deployment Mental Health Assessment was formally codified into law through the FY 2012 NDAA (Pub. L. 112-81, 2011).

In early 2012, DoD Instruction (DoDI) 6490.09 established and specified the roles of the directors of psychological health in each component, both active and reserve. This was an attempt to organize the system and delivery of behavioral health care under an identified point of contact and to incorporate a unified psychological health leadership structure into the Military Health System (MHS). The directors were tasked with coordinating psychological services and ensuring adequate staffing and organizational processes at installations.

Government and Academic Reports

In December 2003, researchers at the Walter Reed Army Institute of Research published the first OIF MHAT report (OIF MHAT, 2003). Its purpose was to improve understanding of behavioral health issues in theater. The team assessed the OIF behavioral health care system by holding several small-group interviews and collecting surveys with 756 soldiers, 82 percent of whom had engaged in combat. Embedding care in forward elements was reported to be useful. Despite inadequate supplies of psychotropic medications, forward-deployed behavioral health teams returned 95 percent of soldiers with behavioral health problems to duty. The researchers found, however, that almost one-half of the service members reported not knowing how to access treatment, and only one-third of those who wanted assistance received it. The report provided recommendations for improving the behavioral health care system.

In 2007, the DoD Task Force on Mental Health published *An Achievable Vision*, which reported that funding and manpower were inadequate to fully support the psychological health of U.S. service members and their families. Following this report, a red cell team was given six months to develop implementation plans for the task force's recommendations. The team worked to improve the culture of military behavioral health care by reducing the stigma of and increasing access to behavioral health services. According to U.S. Government Accountability Office, 2012, p. 8, DoD received more than $2.7 billion to address PTSD and traumatic brain injuries (TBIs) between 2007 and 2010.

Ethics of Operational Psychology

Operational psychologists "apply their skills to operational issues . . . within military, intelligence, transportation, [and] logistics; within special operations; and in support of operators."[1] The primary finding of APA's report on psychological ethics and national security (APA, 2005) was that it is consistent with APA's code of ethics for psychologists to serve as consultants to interrogation or information-gathering processes for national security-related purposes. Stephen H. Behnke, the Director of the APA Office of Ethics, had sponsored that report and was later removed from his position at APA in 2015 after the publication of what is commonly known as the Hoffman Report, which concluded that APA had colluded with DoD to relax the ethical standards for operational psychologists (Hoffman et al., 2015). APA hosts a detailed timeline of events surrounding the ethics of operational psychology (APA, undated), beginning with APA's 1986 statement (reproduced in APA, 2008) condemning torture and subsequent investigations into the actions of DoD, of APA, and congressional inquiries.

---

[1]   Interview with Dr. Carroll Greene, February 11, 2020.

The discussion continues today about the ethical treatment of detainees and psychologists' roles in military operations.

In 2005, DoD Directive 3115.09, *DoD Intelligence Interrogations, Detainee Debriefings, and Tactical Questioning*, provided comprehensive guidance on what behavioral science consultants (BSCs) should and should not do in the context of human intelligence gathering and prohibited them from such activities as providing clinical services for detainees, except in emergencies. Policies governing these practices continue to evolve. In October 2006, the Office of the Surgeon General (OTSG), U.S. Army Medical Command (MEDCOM), released its first formal policies on BSC teams (BSCTs), OTSG/MEDCOM Policy Memo 06-029, *Behavioral Science Consultation Policy*. The memo provided specific guidance on BSCT personnel training requirements, mission, objectives, and authorized and prohibited tasks. The MEDCOM policy mission statement instructed BSCTs to provide psychological expertise and consultation that is "safe, legal, ethical, and effective," with the specific order of qualifiers paralleling the order of values that BSCs were expected to prioritize. The policy also identified categories of personnel that can serve on BSCTs, outlined specific action guidelines for BSCs, and included policy prohibiting certain activities. This policy was later revised and reissued as OTSG/MEDCOM Policy Memo 09-053 and as OTSG/MEDCOM Policy Memo 13-027 (OSTG, 2009; OSTG, 2013).

In June 2006, DoDI 2310.08E, Medical Program Support for Detainee Operations, drew a clear distinction between health care providers who provide behavioral science consultation and those who provide medical, psychological, or behavioral health care and prohibits behavioral science consultants from providing health care or identifying themselves to detainees as providers. It stipulates that behavioral science consultants (BSC) can observe interrogations and advise on detention facilities and environment but may not conduct or direct interrogations.

There continues to be tension between professional ethics and national security needs. In 2006, *Military Psychology* published a special issue on "Operational Psychology and Clinical Practice in Operational Environments," which offered preliminary definitions and roles for an operational psychologist, distinguishing those roles from that of military or combat clinical psychologists. That special issue details the challenges (i.e. ethical, emotional, training) of that role, its demands and complexities. Journal authors called for clear training and practice guidelines to support operational psychologists (Williams and Johnson, 2006).

Organizational Changes

In 2016, Charles Hoge and colleagues published a detailed report on the transformation of the U.S. Army's behavioral health system. Although that report falls outside our time frame, it describes the important changes MEDCOM made to address the behavioral demands of protracted wars that occurred largely between 2003 and 2013. Hoge et al., 2016, describes consolidation of psychiatry, psychology, psychiatric nursing, and social work services under an integrated behavioral health service line; embedding care in brigades; embedding behavioral health providers in primary care; providing routine behavioral health surveillance throughout soldiers' careers; and more.

Some of the transformations in the behavioral health delivery system aimed to reach service members before problems required specialty care. The focus of behavioral health care came to be on prevention and early intervention. Prevention efforts proliferated via resilience-based programs, such as Operational Stress Control and Resilience and Comprehensive Soldier Fitness. Such programs as RESPECT-Mil s(Re-Engineering Systems of Primary Care Treatment in the Military) and the Patient Centered Medical Home were implemented to better recognize (through mandatory screening) and intervene early in the delivery of care for depression and PTSD within primary care to prevent worsening of symptoms that would then require specialty care.

Nevertheless, demand for effective specialty behavioral health care has continued to increase. Emphasis has been on ensuring that all behavioral health providers deliver clinical practice guideline-concurrent care and on building a pipeline of newly trained military psychologists. Measuring the quality of that care is an ongoing challenge. The

Army developed the Behavioral Health Data Portal (BHDP) to deliver self-assessments at intake and in every session so that clinicians can track symptoms in real time and provide feedback to patients. Use of this portal is now required for specialty care assessment and documentation across the services (Defense Health Agency [DHA] Procedural Instruction 6490.02, 2018).

Resources

In January 2004, just as it was becoming clear that OIF would not end quickly and that soldiers were returning with psychological injuries, the first VA/DoD Clinical Practice Guideline for management of PTSD was published. It provided direction for evidenced-based approaches to the assessment and treatment of individuals with PTSD. It became a key source for training military behavioral health providers. In 2010, DoD released Directive Type Memorandum 09-033, *Policy Guidance for Management of Concussion/Mild Traumatic Brain Injury in the Deployed Setting*. Other clinical practice guidelines were published and updated over the 2003–2013 period, one for the treatment of depression and one for the management of concussion. Clinical demand for empirically supported approaches to screening and management of people who are suicidal led to the publication of the first VA/DoD Clinical Practice Guideline for the assessment and management of patients at risk for suicide in June 2013.[2]

---

[2] The guidelines, directives, and other items described in this chapter have been updated periodically since their creation. We are citing only the editions in effect within our time frame.

CHAPTER THREE

Provisioning Military Behavioral Health Care

This chapter describes interviewees' insights regarding provisioning military behavioral health care. Here, *provisioning* includes building, equipping, training, and managing the workforce and the importance of research for tailoring the provision of care.

All but one interview were videotaped. Interviewees signed a release form permitting RAND and the sponsor to use the recordings in the future for education-related activities (see Appendix C). Additional interview material can be found in Appendixes A through D.

The U.S. military was unprepared for a protracted war with significant psychological casualties. The behavioral health system did not have the manpower, structure, or operational strategies needed to respond to the demand for behavioral health services. When Dr. Carl Castro, who was the chief of the Department of Military Psychiatry at the Walter Reed Army Institute of Research and one of our reviewers, described some reasons for this: (1) Immediately following the first Gulf War, the Army's force size was dramatically reduced (from more than 700,000 to just over 400,000); (2) the war was expected not to cost a lot of money or manpower; and (3) the Army had traditionally assessed, diagnosed, and separated soldiers from service so that the VA could treat them. Thus, medical manpower was insufficient, and leaders were disinclined to invest significant funds in behavioral health care at the outset of the wars.

The following sections describe the lessons interviewees believe are important to carry forward.

Manpower

Tools to predict manpower requirements were needed.

Dr. Michael Dinneen, past chairman of the Department of Psychiatry and director of medical services at the National Naval Medical Center (NNMC) in Bethesda, Maryland, said that it took a crisis to direct appropriate manpower to behavioral health needs.[1] Many interviewees spoke about the manpower shortage and the need for hiring. Dr. Eric Getka, National Director for Navy Psychology Training and Recruitment Programs at the time, described one of the challenges with resource management. While he and his team had funds, they were unable to "project the numbers of mental health providers needed and the mix of providers, how many psychiatrists, how many psychologists, how many social workers and so on."[2] Manpower requirements were influenced by the results of the MHATs, which detailed the number and types of providers in theater and the ratio of providers to service members.

Provider Pipelines

It is important to properly incentivize professional psychologist involvement in military careers and to engage human resources early and often in psychologists' career development so that they are aware of and attracted to military careers.

One challenge identified was developing enough interest in military psychology among professional psychologists. Dr. Bruce Crow, who was chief Army psychologist for eight years,[3] discussed building a provider pipeline to address the demand for services. He worked with U.S. Army Recruiting Command and went to various graduate programs to discuss military opportunities for psychologists. He described one challenge in developing a pipeline:

---

[1]   Interview with Dr. Michael Dinneen, April 10, 2020.

[2]   Interview with Dr. Eric Getka, February 11, 2020.

[3]   Interview with Dr. Bruce Crow, August 22, 2019.

Could we create a pipeline that would still attract people from graduate school to come to the Army, knowing that they would really be required to serve longer before they would get their licensure? So, the requirement that [the Army was] seeking was to require licensure before paying back obligated service. Before, it was just completing your internship and then you could start paying back your obligated service.

He said that the Army "ended up being able to get specialty pays and incentive allowances and things like that, analogous to what the psychiatrists were getting. All the things that were necessary for recruiting, retaining, enhancing skills." Crow thought the health professional scholarships helped attract graduate students.

Hiring Practices
DoD requires direct hire authority for behavioral health care specialists to support major overseas contingency operations.

The Uniformed Services University of the Health Sciences (USUHS) medical and clinical psychology doctoral training program produces a fraction of military behavioral health providers; most come from nonmilitary training settings. Interviewees indicated that hiring mechanisms need to be available and efficient. Psychology internship and residency training directors discussed the need to incentivize new hires with the promise of a free education, competitive salaries, and opportunities for deployment.

Three interviewees discussed the regulatory and administrative barriers to hiring. Dr. Mark Paris, past Director of Psychological Health for the Army's Regional Health Command–Atlantic, recalled the challenges associated with hiring more behavioral health providers to meet the demands early in the wars. The U.S. Public Health Service was able to assign providers to DoD, but doing so required a memorandum of agreement between DoD and the U.S. Public Health Service that took more time than preferable to execute.[4] Dr. David Chu, past Under Secretary of Defense for Personnel and Readiness, discussed the

---

[4]   Interview with Dr. Mark Paris, February 12, 2020.

regulatory barriers to hiring DoD civilians. Behavioral health providers were also in high demand in the United States during this period.[5] He explained that not having direct appointing authority from the Office of Personnel Management to hire behavioral health providers hurt DoD's ability to fully staff needed positions. Many providers were not hired because it took so long to do so (and they took other jobs). In 2009, Congress gave DoD direct hire authority for various behavioral health provisions in the law (Pub. L. 110-417, Section 8079). That enabled DoD to build the capacity to better care for service members and families in the military treatment facilities (MTFs) and to decrease wait times by increasing staffing.

Training

Psychologists must be licensed before deploying.

After what were opaquely described as "some unfortunate events" early in the wars, the Army Surgeon General stopped the practice of deploying unlicensed psychologists. Crow and Getka described how the Army and the other services began the practice of assigning psychologists out of internship to a training billet in an MTF for a year (i.e., a residency) to finish their supervised postdoctoral training and become licensed, credentialed psychologists before they could deploy. As noted earlier, this may have been a disincentive for psychologists looking to quickly pay back their education through military service, but it seemed a necessary trade-off.

A single coordinating authority is needed that can prescribe what training and education behavioral health providers should get and how they should get it (institutional training, mobile training, continuing education).

Dr. David Riggs is an instrumental figure in the training of military behavioral health providers. Since 2006, he has operated the CDP, the sponsor of this research, whose mission is to prepare health care professionals to better meet the deployment-related emotional and

---

[5]   Interview with Dr. David Chu, January 8, 2020.

psychological needs of military personnel and their families (CDP, undated). CDP provides a short course for psychology interns, covering such topics as stress and trauma, family, and coping with injuries. CDP also trains civilian providers who may or may not be part of the TRICARE purchased-care network. Civilian providers learn basic terminology and gain exposure to military culture. Early on, CDP found that the providers had different training needs and that the intensity, location, and topics of training needed to be adjusted. For instance, CDP initially conducted a three-week short course at USUHS; that soon became a two-week course. CDP ultimately brought the training directly to the MTFs, offering training in evidenced-based treatment approaches, such as prolonged exposure and cognitive processing therapy. The organization of the military education system posed some challenges for CDP, because it is part of the USUHS and not affiliated with the U.S. Army Medical Department Center and School.[6] This meant that CDP was largely excluded from education planning that could be delivered in coordination with and that better aligned with traditional military training programs.

Dr. David Orman, past Chief of Psychiatry at Brooke Army Medical Center, said that education lags developments in practice.[7] And as Riggs conveyed, it is difficult to adjust a curriculum in the middle of a multiyear training program. Thus, curricula cannot be as flexible as may be necessary in fast-changing environments. This is more reason to learn from the past and anticipate the future when training the workforce.

Operational Psychology

Operational psychologists need clear guidance on adherence to ethical practices within their operational support roles.

Dr. Carroll Greene was the first psychologist assigned to several special mission units within Joint Special Operations Command, from

---

[6]   The Army Medical Department Center and School officially changed its name to "U.S. Army Medical Center of Excellence," or MEDCoE, effective Sunday, September 15, 2019.

[7]   Interview with Dr. David Orman, April 14, 2020.

1998 through 2004.[8] He described the role of the military operational psychologist that predominantly developed within Special Forces as applying "their skills to operational issues . . . within military, intelligence, transportation, logistics, within special operations and in support of operators."[9] Operational psychologists may support threat assessment, interrogation, other intelligence activities, and counterespionage and may train operators and intelligence professionals to be effective at getting information. Greene was involved in developing the first set of guidelines governing the practice of operational psychology. He said he and some other psychologists attending the annual Survival, Evasion, Resistance and Escape conference consulted with Stephen H. Behnke, director of the APA's Office of Ethics, to ensure that the guidelines met APA's ethical standards. Significant controversy followed, with accusations that DoD was using psychologists to support enhanced interrogation activities. The ethical standards and practices for psychologists in various detainee care or interrogation situations are still being developed today.

In Chapter Two, we described some of the DoD policies that have evolved as tension between professional ethics and national security needs continues. Greene pointed out that 99 percent of the APA members that voted on what constitutes ethical practices for operational psychologists had never been in the military themselves and did not "know about the mindset or the ethics of military operational psychologists."[10] He went on to address the challenges of coordination of roles of the psychologists delivering care and those supporting operational needs:

> So, you've got one psychologist supporting health care of the guard force, the administration, as well as the detainees. You've got another psychologist supporting just the operational interrogational side of it. Then, who can do what? Can the clinical psychologist let the operational psychologist know anything about

---

[8]   Interview with Dr. Carroll Greene, February 11, 2020.

[9]   Interview with Dr. Carroll Greene, February 11, 2020.

[10]   Interview with Dr. Carroll Greene, February 11, 2020.

some disorder, or dysfunction, or physical, or mental need that a detainee has?[11]

The negotiation of ethical practices within national security contexts is complex. We interviewed one expert on this, Greene. Many other opinions and details need to be captured to derive more specific lessons. For more information, APA maintains a detailed timeline of events and policy statements (APA, undated).

Locations and Assignments

Embedded behavioral health care is critical for establishing rapport, early intervention, and effective care. Providers need to be prepared to operate as organic assets, assigned to a unit, and to communicate their value and role to commanders and service members.

The interviewees all believed that embedding behavioral health care in units and in primary care was a game changer. Most interviewees addressed embedded care in some way, with the belief that proximity to troops matters for building trust and access. Dr. Rebecca Porter, past Army Director of Psychological Health, described differences in how behavioral health care was embedded during wartime: *organic* personnel were assigned to units, *attached* personnel were assigned to an MTF. As she explained,

> embedded behavioral health is a concept that refers to almost like a behavioral health clinic in the brigade garrison area. What some people mean when they say embedded behavioral health is *organic*, and organic behavioral health is when you've got them assigned to the unit. They are uniformed soldiers. You've got a psychologist or social worker or behavioral health tech that is actually assigned to the brigade and they call them BHOs, Behavioral Health Officers. They're assigned to the brigade. They train with the brigade. They go downrange with the brigade.

---

[11] Interview with Dr. Carroll Greene, February 11, 2020.

She stated that the two programs, one for embedded and one for organic providers, were added to the TO&E [table of organization and equipment].[12]

CDR Robert Lippy, who was the officer in charge of the Combat Stress Clinic at Camp Dwyer, Helmand Province, in 2010, described differences in the types of deployments, depending on how embedded the providers were. As he explained,

> I deployed with a medical battalion, and so we deployed as companies, two separate companies out of that Marine Corps medical battalion. So, basically, what it does is [that] it takes what they call health service augmentation personnel, basically personnel from the MTFs, and they're given TAD [temporary additional duty] orders to med[ical] battalions where they then deployed again for that deployment.

Getka explained that the Navy began putting psychologists on aircraft carriers in the 1990s.[13] He said that commanders embraced having a psychologist in operating environments because the number of medevacs off the ships for behavioral health care dropped to almost zero. However, early in OIF, psychologists that deployed on ships came out of Navy hospitals, having trained in a medical model that was not a good fit for the operational environment that they were being thrown into. He went on to say that an early challenge for psychologists operating in combat environments was that they did not know how to describe their value proposition, "This is what I'm here to do, this is what I can do." Getka believes that the shift to the operational stress control (nonmedical) model reliant on a stress continuum is what enabled psychologists to better communicate with sailors and with commands.

---

[12] Interview with Dr. Rebecca Porter, January 31, 2020.

[13] Interview with Dr. Eric Getka, February 11, 2020.

Equipping

Providers need to know the contents of and how to use the latest clinical practice guidelines and assessment instruments as these tools continue to evolve.

Behavioral health providers' equipment includes clinical tools for assessment (screeners and questionnaires) and treatment methods (clinical guidelines for evidence-based practice). The first VA/DoD clinical practice guideline for the treatment of acute stress disorder and PTSD was published in 2004. This guideline evaluated the clinical research, described the level of evidence for each intervention, and recommended empirically supported practices; it prescribed best practices for behavioral health providers to follow when treating traumatic stress.

Validated screening tools and questionnaires were recommended to identify depression, PTSD, general anxiety, and suicidality. These instruments allowed behavioral health providers to understand an individual's symptoms and offered a way of communicating with patients about their health. Screening questionnaires for PTSD, depression, suicidality, and substance abuse have established psychometric properties and do not require clinician judgement to score them. It is more difficult to assess TBI in a war zone.[14]

Research

Efforts to streamline and reduce the time required for regulatory review of behavioral health studies could bring health solutions to service members sooner.

Interviewees from a variety of backgrounds and roles noted the need for better, faster, and more innovative research. What was common across interviewees was frustration—with the pace of research, with the extent to which research drives program implemen-

---

[14] Phone conversation with Dr. James Kelly, past director of the National Intrepid Center of Excellence.

tation, and with what GEN Peter Chiarelli, past Vice Chief of Staff of the Army, described as an incentive system that impedes progress because of competition among researchers and because of the drive for academic tenure. Chiarelli said that "people need to sit down and say how do we change the incentive system to get us working together [toward a common goal]."[15]

Maintaining a cohesive research infrastructure such that baseline data are continuously collected will enable a quicker response to research demands in the next war. Research on DoD health services has evolved, and programs typically collect some form of program evaluation. Dinneen said, "It takes a war to innovate."[16] Innovation requires evaluation. Efforts to standardize and evaluate programs reflected the military's cultural shift to evidence-based practice. Research is necessary to address the next health concern, but research lags clinical needs and practices. That led to some untested programs being implemented without an evaluation component to assess outcomes. Research is also expensive. It was not until 2007 that substantial resources were allocated to study military mental health.

Terri Tanielian, a senior scientist at RAND, addressed her experiences conducting two large studies of service member and family health. Regulatory review of DoD research is time consuming and comes with constraints. Tanielian described having to go through DoD regulatory requirements,

> which meant that our sampling approach as well as our survey instrument had to go through their review. During that process, we were advised that it would not be approved if it included anything about substance use or anything about military sexual harassment or sexual assault. So, we removed those items. [17]

These barriers to research impede the development of new knowledge and solutions that could improve the lives of service

---

[15] Interview with GEN Peter Chiarelli, April 15, 2020.

[16] Interview with Dr. David Orman, April 10, 2020.

[17] Interview with Terri Tanielian, February 20, 2020.

members and their families. The assessment of sensitive topics, such as mental health, in human subjects research is heavily scrutinized and regulated. Thus, it was difficult to conduct research on PTSD and substance abuse and evaluate of treatment programs and publish in a timely fashion. This delayed programmatic changes that could have brought more effective care to service members sooner. DoD has worked to improve the research infrastructure and reduce review time, but the problem remains.

Chapter Summary

Manpower shortfalls made it difficult to meet the demand for behavior health services—with problems stemming both from the inability to estimate requirements and difficulty accessing providers. Interviewees discussed obstacles and solutions for building a provider pipeline (using scholarships, retention bonuses, and other financial incentives) and for hiring the needed number and mix of providers. It seemed the big lesson interviewees described is that it is possible to surge to meet new demands on the behavioral health system, but there need to be avenues for hiring and appropriate incentives to do so. Interviewees described several lessons about provisioning behavioral health care between 2003 and 2013:

- Tools to predict manpower requirements were needed.
- It is important to properly incentivize professional psychologist involvement in military careers and to engage human resources early and often in psychologists' career development so that they are aware of and attracted to military careers.
- DoD requires direct-hire authority for behavioral health care specialists to support major overseas contingency operations. Psychologists must be licensed before deploying.
- A single coordinating authority is needed that can prescribe what training and education behavioral health providers should get and the modality (institutional training, mobile training, continuing education) by which they should get it. Operational psychologists

need clear guidance on adherence to ethical practices within their operational support roles.

- Embedded behavioral health care is critical for establishing rapport, early intervention, and effective care.
- Providers need to be prepared to operate as organic assets, assigned to a unit, and to communicate their value and role to commanders and service members.
- Providers need to know the contents of and how to use the latest clinical practice guidelines and assessment instruments as these tools continue to evolve.
- Efforts to streamline and reduce the time required for regulatory review of behavioral health studies could bring health solutions to service members sooner.

CHAPTER FOUR

Delivery of Military Behavioral Health Care

Behavioral health services are quite varied, including prevention, early intervention, health monitoring, and treatment (of service members, spouses, and children). Provider roles are quite varied as well. The interviewees described important changes to the health system that affected the delivery of care and discussed behavioral health within the care delivery system, the roles, the models under which providers practiced, and the electronic systems for documenting care delivery.

Organization of the Military Behavioral Health Care System

Behavioral health providers need to be prepared to practice in MTFs, in theater, and in different roles, depending on the setting (i.e., primary care, specialty care, and consultation).

The behavioral health system underwent massive change over the first decade of OIF and OEF. Crow said that, between 2003 and 2005,

> the Army transition to brigade-oriented configuration was maturing, so we had more psychologists going into brigades as the brigade behavioral health officer. Social workers were also in those positions. But our psychologists, and this is where we were training them to be comfortable going into a brigade able to provide consultation to a brigade commander, a battalion commander, a company commander, and not only be focused on clinical work with one patient at a time but to think organizationally about,

how do you advise a commander in a way that makes sense to him or her, of what can they do at the organizational level and in their leadership role.[1]

The Army also transformed the way behavioral health was delivered by forming the Behavioral Health Service Line, which included social work, psychology, and psychiatry departments, instead of each operating separately. The intent was to remove stovepipes in behavioral health disciplines and to improve continuity of care (Hoge et al., 2016). The idea was there was "no wrong door" when seeking behavioral health support.[2] This led to treatment teams delivering care, and Orman said that any member of the treatment team could lead the team,[3] meaning that there was no natural hierarchy by discipline. He said,

> the psychiatrist typically is not the team lead. So any issues of who's the authority, who's leading the team, et cetera, by design, we made sure that was specialty non-dependent. And that, in essence we wanted the team to operate as a team and do what they uniquely do well from their various specialty vantage points, to contribute to the welfare of the soldiers that were accessing the team for treatment.[4]

The Army's combat stress control doctrine was in development and aimed to organize care based on need, not function. Crow said,

> One of the things that I think was the major shift in doctrine was, the Army combat stress control doctrine was built around the notion that you had kind of segregated functions, primarily in prevention versus treatment. And there was a configuration, there were treatment teams, prevention teams, and there were functions associated with those, but they were segregated. And

---

[1]   Interview with Dr. Bruce Crow, August 22, 2019.

[2]   Interview with Dr. Michael Dinneen, April 10, 2020.

[3]   Interview with Dr. David Orman, April 10, 2020.

[4]   Interview with Dr. David Orman, April 10, 2020.

one thing that we saw in theater was, it just wasn't logical at all, a soldier who was close to a prevention team, and that was the only behavioral health support in the area, went to the local behavioral health people that were in their area to ask for services, and that team would say, "Well, we don't do treatment. We only do prevention. You'll have to go to some other location." It was a drive, it was in an unsecure area, and it just kind of didn't make sense. So that type of experience and observation led to a shift in doctrine that every behavioral health provider was a combat and operational stress control officer. Every provider. And they would need to know all of the functions and be able to deliver all the functions based on need—so, not based on the role that you were assigned within the unit, [but] based on need of the organization you were supporting based on the need of the soldiers that were receiving support. So that was a pretty big shift in thinking about doctrine and, again, the training that would be needed for personnel and then how to deliver it, how to organize the services.[5]

A center of excellence for behavioral health needs to be empowered to coordinate services within the MHS.

Another important development in the organization of care was the establishment of the Defense Centers of Excellence for Psychological Health and Traumatic Brain Injury (DCoE) in 2007. DCoE was charged with ensuring excellence in behavioral health care, a broad mission that encompassed education, outreach, training, and research to further the effectiveness of psychological health care. However, DCoE existed outside the health delivery system. It was a large agency, with a large mission, and the centers "built the plane while flying it."[6] Dr. Charles Engel, past director of the DoD Deployment Health Clinical Center, explained:

The operations of the health system were the responsibility of the services, the Army, Navy, Air Force, [and] marines, and the

---

[5]   Interview with Dr. Bruce Crow, August 22, 2019.

[6]   Interview with Dr. Charles Engel, February 17, 2020.

> DoD piece was policy so there was this huge policy shop [DCoE], and they were receiving tremendous resources, and I think there was a sense on the part of the provider community and the services that . . . the money was going there and not getting used appropriately.[7]

In 2013, DCoE was reorganized, and different components moved to DHA, which was established in October 2013 to consolidate the service MTFs into a triservice health system. That meant that Army, Navy, and Air Force behavioral health providers would need to adjust to new workflows and procedures. Efforts to standardize procedures and documentation affected providers' work experiences and feelings about work. Engel said,

> One might hope that, with the unification of the system under DHA, that an activity like DCoE, if stood up in a future conflict, may be in a better place to be operationally connected, but it was disconnected in some ways that it couldn't really help . . . it was a structural organizational flaw in many ways.[8]

Models of Behavioral Health Care

Nonmedical Model

Behavioral health providers need to be prepared to address prevention and health within a nonmedical model.

The military's extensive efforts to reduce behavioral health stigma as a barrier to care included shifts away from a medical model to a nonmedical model that focused on prevention of symptoms outside the clinical setting instead of the treatment of clinical disorders. To reduce stigma and encourage behavioral health care–seeking, a stress continuum model and efforts to normalize PTSD as a normal reaction to abnormal circumstances ensued. Providers need to buy into this

---

[7] Interview with Dr. Charles Engel, February 17, 2020.

[8] Interview with Dr. Charles Engel, February 17, 2020.

approach and learn to convey it to service members and commanders as needed.

Providers need to capably deliver prevention practices (i.e., pre-clinical activities, such as resilience-building, psychoeducation, stress management). According to Dr. William Nash, past director of psychological health for the U.S. Marine Corps, the stress continuum is important in operational stress control (such as the Operational Stress Control and Resilience model) and for communicating with service members and line leadership.[9] The training most behavioral health providers receive involves recognizing, diagnosing, and treating psychopathology. Psychology training typically does not focus on the prevention of disorders, except for early intervention to prevent long-term impairment, so prevention is a new skill psychologists need.

Patient-Centered Medical Home

Integration of behavioral and nonbehavioral health care is critical. Behavioral health providers need to be prepared to practice in the primary-care setting.

In the MTF, behavioral health providers (technicians, counselors, and psychologists) are on-site resources in primary care; this is the Patient-Centered Medical Home model. Over the past decade, the MHS has worked to implement a collaborative care model in which patients are the hub and in which providers work together as a unit caring for the patient. The military worked to transform primary-care delivery, to improve care coordination, continuity, and quality. Engel said, "primary care is the backbone of care. It's where the service members are being seen and it's really where the greatest need was."[10] He indicated that a crucial aspect of the Patient-Centered Medical Home model is the universal screening that occurs during every visit to primary care. Behavioral health screening tools can quickly determine whether it would be useful to involve the on-site care manager or inte-

---

[9]   Interview with Dr. William Nash, February 20, 2020.

[10]   Interview with Dr. Charles Engel, February 17, 2020.

grated behavioral health provider. That provider can deliver short-term care and determine whether a referral to specialty care is needed.[11]

Prevention: Health Screening and Resilience-Building

Behavioral health providers need to capably deliver prevention and psychoeducation activities and conduct routine health surveillance.

The lessons of the first Gulf War did not lead the MHS to anticipate the medical needs of the new wars. These lessons did, however, teach the military the importance of health surveillance. As Tanielian stated, "one of the big lessons of the first Gulf war, was really kind of defining and paving the way for our postdeployment health assessment so that we were trying to monitor for some of those concerns."[12] Mandatory health screening is crucial. Routine health assessments—annually, predeployment, postdeployment, and three to six months postdeployment—are essential ways to track individual health status and to bring service members into contact with the health system. The FY 2007 NDAA added the requirement for service members to have face-to-face meetings with behavioral health providers when reviewing the health assessments (Pub. L. 109-36, 2006). This was important both for health monitoring and for offering service members an experience with a behavioral health provider.

Tanielian also spoke about people's expectations: "If we could just improve resilience or we can improve readiness, that would mitigate some of these [health] consequences."[13] Interviewees expressed varied opinions about the value of resilience-building programs. Chu viewed them as necessary but not effective enough; he suggested that research is needed to compare resilience-building approaches to develop effective strategies.[14] Clinicians expressed skepticism about the military's expectation that negative psychological sequelae of war could be

---

[11] Interview with Dr. Charles Engel, February 17, 2020.

[12] Interview with Terri Tanielian, February 20, 2020.

[13] Interview with Terri Tanielian, February 20, 2020.

[14] Interview with Dr. David Chu, January 8, 2020.

mitigated through resilience training. In fact, some suggested that the shift to prevention sent the wrong message to troops—implying that postwar behavioral health problems could (or should) be prevented.

GEN (ret.) Eric Schoomaker, past Army Surgeon General, said it was GEN George Casey who pressed him for a solution to prevent people from "drifting over that line" from stress into impairment.[15] Schoomaker believes that is where to focus the Battlemind program to prevent deployment and postdeployment problems. The Battlemind program (Adler et al., 2009) has many components, most of which are taught by behavioral health providers. Psychoeducation, such as teaching people to recognize behavioral health symptoms, is one essential component. The Battlemind program is intended to prepare service members for the stress of deployment and to assist service members with redeployment adjustments. Orman said that the program reflected the Army's move away from a medical model of psychological disorders (which focuses on pathology and treatment) toward a nonmedical approach to preventing stress and normalizing stress reactions. This was consistent with the Marine Corps' reliance on the stress continuum.

Command Consultation

Behavioral health providers need to be able to articulate their role and value to commanders, understand confidentiality policies, and communicate the minimum necessary information to address the information commanders need to know to maintain unit readiness.

Behavioral health providers often determine fitness for duty, and commanders rely on these providers for feedback on an individual's readiness. That requires providers to maintain a relationship with service members and with their "bosses." Porter said she discussed this idea of dual agency and having "two masters" as early as internship. She

---

[15] Interview with LTG Dr. Eric Schoomaker, April 17, 2020.

thought it was possible in most cases "to navigate that in a respectful, ethical way."[16]

Many interviewees described the importance of being able to articulate the value and role of the behavioral health provider (either embedded in units or in garrison). Ensuring providers can communicate effectively with both service members and commanders about the value and capabilities of the health provider is important. Lippy indicated that one of the bigger changes in care delivery during the wars was the emphasis on communication with line commanders. Although that was always an important role for behavioral health providers, Lippy said, "there's just been increasing emphasis on that as really the standard of care."[17] DoDI 6490.08, 2011, provides guidance on what information should be provided to satisfy the purpose of a disclosure. Lippy indicated "that [the DoDI] specifies that balance of confidentiality with a commander's need to know, so who's ultimately responsible for his sailors, and marines. So, it outlines those nine conditions of when you not only can break confidentiality, but you're actually required to do that."[18]

Treatment

Behavioral health providers need to be trained to follow VA/DoD clinical practice guidelines for the treatment of PTSD, depression, and other psychological disorders in service members and their families and to document their practices.

The prevalence of war-related PTSD, depression, and TBI placed great demand on the behavioral health delivery system. The first edition of the VA/DoD clinical practice guideline for PTSD was issued in 2004, around the time awareness of postcombat adjustment and behavioral health problems became a focus of the new wars in Iraq and Afghanistan (Management of Post-Traumatic Stress Working

---

[16] Interview with Dr. Rebecca Porter, January 31, 2020.

[17] Interview with CDR Robert Lippy, August 22, 2019.

[18] Interview with CDR Robert Lippy, August 22, 2019.

Group, 2004). These guidelines offered providers an evidence-based roadmap to the assessment and treatment of PTSD. Psychologists were then trained to deliver manualized cognitive behavioral therapy to service members in garrison. Manualized therapies have explicit instructions for what care to deliver when and for how to measure symptom improvements. Standardized treatment approaches that rely on measurement-based interventions are conducive to quality assessment. The MHS had ramped up and transformed to meet the demands of the wars, and providers were adjusting to the growing interest in the effectiveness of their services. Providers needed to accept that care delivery was standardized, manualized, and scrutinized.

In the theater of war, clinical care focused on assessment and treatment planning. The job of assets organic to the infantry units was "to be closer to the battlefront where they would do sort of a unit circulation. So, go around and sort of talk to the troops probably a little bit more similar to like what a chaplain does."[19]

Behavioral health providers need to be prepared to document care delivery using standardized tools conducive to measuring the quality of their care.

The evolution of the electronic medical record and the Armed Forces Health Longitudinal Technology Application–Theater enabled deployed providers to document care in low-communication environments. Lippy was surprised by the ease of medical charting in theater. He said that

> it was amazing that, here we are, we're in the middle of a desert at this base. It was built from scratch, and I had a laptop, and I was able to connect to electronic medical records. It was primarily a push system. So, I could enter my notes, which would go into the big electronic medical record. A little bit more challenging, though, [was] pulling information. So, if I had to review patient's records, it was a little bit more challenging to get that informa-

---

[19] Interview with CDR Robert Lippy, August 22, 2019.

tion. I was able to get it, it just, it was a little bit of a lag with it and it wasn't always a reliable system that was up.[20]

A crucial advancement in understanding the effectiveness of behavioral health care was the development of the BHDP. It was built to capture patient-level data, to facilitate screening and measurement-based care via symptom assessments, and to guide clinicians in delivering measurement-based care. It has enabled the reporting of key metrics about response to treatment and quality of care and the evaluation of treatment patterns and response. Medical record documentation and use of the BHDP are important for measuring the quality of care. As Dr. Jonathan Woodson, past Assistant Secretary of Defense for Health Affairs, said,

> it was about building those information systems that could track therapies that soldiers, sailors, airmen, and marines were receiving; the effects of those therapies; and then again, track it over time and space for [an] iterative sort of advancement. But also, at the individual level, to make sure that individuals were responding and weren't lost in the cracks, so to speak, as [they] transfer from duty station to duty station or from military service to civilian life.[21]

Families need support through multiple and frequent deployment cycles.

Porter described being an assistant to GEN Eric Shinseki on September 11, 2001. She recalled that it was Shinseki's wife who immediately drew attention to the needs of families. It was her experience as an Army spouse during Vietnam that underscored the importance of caring for families while warfighters are deployed.[22] Tanielian thought that

---

[20] Interview with CDR Robert Lippy, August 22, 2019.

[21] Interview with Dr. Jonathan Woodson, April 17, 2020.

[22] Interview with Dr. Rebecca Porter, January 31, 2020.

one of the lessons from previous deployments is that, when a service member serves, the family serves. There's the social contract that is implicit with the relationship that the services and the DoD have with the troops, that they take care of their families. And so there was a desire to serve them, but there wasn't necessarily a lot of research to inform the needs.[23]

Military beneficiaries (spouses and children of service members) seek care in MTFs, and adult and child behavioral health providers need to be capable of delivering effective care to them. Research on the family members' need for support and an emphasis in military health care on behavioral health led to many behavioral support programs for service members' spouses and children (for example, Military OneSource, Military Family Life Counselors, and the Yellow Ribbon program). The frequency of deployments placed significant strains on the family, and deployment schedules were unlike those for any prior war. Efforts continue to understand the best ways to support military families.

In retrospect, we should have asked our experts more about behavioral health policies for spouses and children. Only two experts raised families as a topic of discussion. We did not sufficiently address the lessons learned about caring for beneficiaries, and that remains an important topic for further study.

Chapter Summary

Interviewees offered several lessons about the delivery of military behavioral health care based on their experiences:

- Behavioral health providers need to be prepared to practice in MTFs, in theater, and in different roles, depending on the setting (i.e., primary care, specialty care, and consultation).
- A center of excellence for behavioral health needs to be empowered to coordinate services within the MHS.

---

[23] Interview with Terri Tanielian, February 20, 2020.

- Behavioral health providers need to be prepared to address prevention and health within a nonmedical model. Integration of behavioral and nonbehavioral health care is critical. Behavioral health providers need to be prepared to practice in the primary-care setting.
- It is important for military behavioral health providers to be effective assessment technicians during all touch points and to feel competent delivering preclinical interventions to build resilience among the military population.
- Behavioral health providers need to be able to articulate their role and value to commanders, understand confidentiality policies, and communicate the minimum necessary information to address the information commanders need to know to maintain unit readiness.
- Behavioral health providers need to be trained to follow VA/DoD clinical practice guidelines for the treatment of PTSD, depression, and other psychological disorders in service members and their families.
- Behavioral health providers need to be prepared to document care delivery using standardized tools conducive to measuring the quality of their care.
- Families need support through multiple and frequent deployment cycles.

CHAPTER FIVE

Reflections

In this chapter, we reflect broadly on what changed between 2003 and 2013 and whether the changes were helpful. We offer some ideas for future efforts to build on the lessons we began collecting here.

Where Did We Begin?

Many interviewees felt compelled to describe the history of military behavioral health care in the first Gulf War, after the Pentagon attack on 9/11, and the Anthrax attacks following 9/11. Chu reported an increased focus on behavioral health in late 2001.[1] After 9/11, Operation Solace was implemented, which was "therapy by walking around."[2] The need for an immediate behavioral health response the weeks and months after 9/11 led to the development of this model of care: bringing stress management and other counseling to the individual, instead of waiting for people to present in a formal health care setting. Thus, Operation Solace was viewed as a precursor to the embedded behavioral health model.

In the first Gulf War, medically unexplained physical symptoms became the pressing health concern, and research expanded to understand and mitigate such symptoms. PTSD and TBI were not high priorities at the time. After 9/11, the military and the public expected a

---

[1]   Interview with Dr. David Chu, January 8, 2020.

[2]   Interview with Dr. Charles Engel, February 17, 2020; Interview with Dr. Dave Orman, April 14, 2020.

"quick" war similar to the first Gulf War, which lasted three weeks in 1991. The behavioral health system was stovepiped within MTFs. Psychiatry, psychology, and social work were three separate departments. There were no DoD clinical practice guidelines for treating PTSD. Medical surveillance was in place, however. As Tanielian indicated, one lesson of the first Gulf War was the importance of medical surveillance.[3]

Where Did We Go?

The establishment of the Army's behavioral health service line removed the stovepipes and merged the behavioral health disciplines to improve the coordination of behavioral health care (Hoge et al., 2016). To overcome barriers to behavioral health care utilization, providers were often assigned to line units, deploying with their units, and often operated outside the wire (the perceived safety of the secured forward operating base). The medical model of behavioral health care shifted to a stress continuum model that resonated with line leaders and service members. This included resilience-building efforts aimed at preventing the downstream consequences of trauma exposure. The periodic health assessment and other surveillance and screening efforts became well established, with revised procedures to emphasize behavioral health symptom assessment and provider contact.

What Worked?

The answers derive from interviewees' beliefs. We did not conduct a literature review or structured data analysis to establish the effectiveness of each of the key policy shifts. Instead, we report on the perceptions of the senior leaders we interviewed. Interviewees believed surveillance and the reliance on research to drive clinical practice improved behavioral health care. Surveillance (using the MHATs and mandatory health

---

[3]   Interview with Terri Tanielian, February 20, 2020.

screening) enabled the military to understand population health needs to determine provider staffing needs. Empirically supported screening and intervention techniques enabled recognition of those in need of behavioral health care. Providers were trained to follow VA/DoD clinical practice guidelines, embedded care, and collaborative care. The BHDP was developed by the Army. It is such an important workflow and quality management tool that it is now used across services to electronically capture behavioral health symptom and treatment data to drive care and facilitate the evaluation of care quality.

What Did Not Work?

Knowledge of what works and what does not is lacking in most areas. For example, the effectiveness of resilience-building and suicide-prevention efforts remains largely unknown, partly because of the challenges of conducting controlled research on these topics and partly because of a lack of resources for program evaluation. It is also challenging to assess the value of health system changes in terms of cost and quality. Thus, until there is careful quantitative assessment of major policy and organizational changes, we will not know how effective the changes were.

Interviewees agreed that policy changes were generally reactive rather than proactive. They described a variety of frustrating experiences and events. The FY 2007 congressional allocation of $900 million in a budgetary supplement was necessary but led to pressure for quick, instead of thoughtful, spending. The establishment of a center of excellence was generally viewed as a good idea, but the establishment of DCoE was problematic. DCoE had an ambitious mission but was not organizationally empowered to change practice.

Dinneen said it was problematic that so much innovation without evaluation followed significant increases in available funding. He suggested the MHS should be able to surge by increasing all it is already doing: "Don't do special stuff; do the stuff you were already doing, but do it right."[4]

Next Steps

This effort to understand important lessons that were learned in the face of intense demands from high-OPTEMPO wars in Iraq and Afghanistan just scratches the surface of what may be valuable takeaways from the past several decades of operational experience. Certainly, there are more lessons to learn about such a high-profile and complex topic as the provision of behavioral care during OIF and OEF. We hope this effort spurs other efforts to capture important lessons.

We sidestepped the politics behind the wars; for example, how the views of the general public affected service members' experiences, how line commanders managed resources needed for the wars, and what the commanders expected the capabilities of the behavioral health workforce to be. As Kieran's book jacket says, the military mental health crisis "is the story of how medical conditions intersect with larger political questions about militarism and foreign policy" (Kieran, 2019). We hope that researchers and historians will build on this work to include more in-depth analysis of specific policy changes, to understand lessons stemming from political controversies, and to cover a longer period. Our goal is for the lessons reported here to drive questions for further research. For example, deeper examination of events occurring from 2013 to the present may reveal important lessons about how troop reductions and changing OPTEMPO have affected the behavioral health system or how past lessons may be applied to a changing battlefield. The categories we imposed on the interviewee's insights may provide a useful structure for future efforts to capture additional lessons learned.

---

[4]   Interview with Dr. Michael Dinneen, April 10, 2020.

Conclusions

The findings stemming from this effort to understand lessons from the complex and fluid events surrounding the delivery of behavioral health care from 2003 through 2013 can be viewed as research questions in need of evaluation. Our work is subjective. We selected the events that seemed most important, selected the interviewees, (largely) selected the interview topics, and selected interview excerpts from a wealth of material the experts provided. Subsequent researchers repeating this process would likely derive different takeaways from another group of events and experts.

The depth of the expertise captured and the range of topics discussed are not easily synthesized. Interview questions were open ended, and interviewees brought unique perspectives while recalling events and causal relationships. Thus, the interview audio and video files offer a legacy from which to derive further insights. The files, which have been transcribed, are an important project deliverable for CDP, which plans to mine the transcripts to understand specific topics, events, and lessons. These chapters really scratch the surface of the input we received. Interviewees discussed topics other than the provision and delivery of military behavioral health care; for instance, several interviewees described the importance of standardized program implementation procedures. We excluded such topics when selecting interview excerpts.

It is also important to evaluate the lessons described here. Further research on the effectiveness of the responses to evolving behavioral health demands is warranted. Research on the effectiveness of embedded care delivery models, training programs, and quality of care may validate the opinions of the experts we interviewed. Some interviewees pointed out that better anticipating events, being proactive instead of reactive, is critical going forward. As Getka put it, "looking back is extremely valuable, but trying to look forward to anticipate what the psychological needs of the future warfighter are going to be is just as important."[5]

---

[5] Interview with Dr. Eric Getka, February 11, 2020.

Interview Procedures

The lead author (Gore) emailed potential interviewees a request for an on-the-record interview and conducted all the interviews. Interviewees signed a release (see Appendix C) to allow RAND to record the audio and video content for CDP for the purpose of educating audiences. Interviews lasted approximately 90 minutes. Three interviews were conducted in person in the RAND studio; one was conducted by telephone; and the remainder were conducted using the Zoom video meeting platform, which enabled video screens to be pinned to the interviewee and interview content be easily transcribed. We drew inferences from the timeline of events we developed for CDP regarding the most significant topics or themes represented. Identifying these themes was largely subjective and intuitive. We developed a priori categories for the timeline (policies, ethics of operational psychology, government reports, organizational change, academic literature, and resources and training tools). We considered an event to have high impact if it was something that altered clinical practice *and* if the interviewees addressed it. We asked ourselves whether these downstream changes would have occurred if the event had not occurred. We also assumed that the high-profile events are connected to policy and system changes.

Selection of Interviewees

We aimed to ensure expert coverage of each major event when selecting interviewees. Interviewees were selected because of their experiences with the important events during the 2003–2013 period. In addition, we considered the following factors: professional role, branch of service, period of service, and influence on development and implementation of key policies. We aimed to identify a cohort that covered broad topic areas during different periods in OIF and OEF from different echelons of leadership, including line and medical leaders. We reviewed task force participants, policy signatories, and directors of psychological health and relied on expert opinion and snowball sampling. We asked specific military researchers and clinicians for recommendations. Interviewees recommended other individuals to address certain topics. We maintained a list of approximately 42 potential interviewees. Our goal was to reach up to 20 individuals who could address one or many topics we considered important to the provision and delivery of military behavioral health care. Eleven people declined or did not respond to our invitation. We tried to find alternate interviewees to address topics when individuals declined, although gaps remain in the final sample. We are missing social workers, behavioral health technicians, and congressional policymakers.

Interview Outreach

We identified potential interviewee candidates based on the events and themes observed in the timeline. We emailed an interview request tailored to the experiences of the selected experts. We provided a brief explanation of the study and interview plan. We offered the interviewee a primer to evoke thoughts about a variety of topics included in CDP's purview regarding the provision and delivery of military behavioral health care (see Appendix B).

Interview Approach

The interview goals were defined, but the content was open ended and dictated by the interviewees. Thus, we can describe our structured methods, but they are not replicable. We did not adhere to a strict interview protocol; instead, we aimed to follow the ideas raised during the interview. We asked policymakers different questions from those we asked clinicians in each service branch. We approached each interview testing the idea that system and training changes were reactive. We aimed to understand the drivers of change, different courses of action considered before implementing change, experiences and hindsight. Essentially, the question was this: "If you knew then what you know now, what would you have done differently."

Information from early interviews informed both the selection and content of later interviews. While knowledge of major events in the timeline influenced the interviewer prompts, interviewees were asked to describe the lessons they learned and highlight the topics they considered themselves best equipped to address. Interviewees tended to have had long military careers with many different commands and roles. They brought the expertise and determined the topics discussed, while the interviewer maintained some structure and focus on how these lessons applied to behavioral health providers.

Interview Protocol

The following is the protocol that we provided to the interviewees to evoke their ideas about key lessons learned. It was edited slightly to focus on the interviewees' specific areas of expertise.

Project goal: To identify lessons learned from OIF/OEF for preparing behavioral health providers for future conflicts.

Interview goals: Understand the rationale for major policy, structural, and other changes in the delivery of military behavioral health care and highlight key events and eras in military psychological and behavioral health care during OEF/OIF.

> ** **What lessons were learned about delivering behavioral health care during OIF/OEF that should be carried forward for any future conflicts?** **

Primary Questions

What would you change about the mental health delivery system? Why? Based on what experience? What information was needed to identify the problem and institute changes in the system?

Prompts and Follow-On Questions

- Describe events or issues that forced change.
- Describe significant changes in policy or practice. Include any major turning points or "new eras" that occur to you.
  - How did changes in policy affect practice? And vice versa?
  - Assess those changes—were they good/bad, would there have been a better direction/plan to address specific issues in behavioral health?
  - What adaptations were prompted by these changes?

Potential Practitioner Topic Areas

- preparation, education, self-care
- outreach, screening, intake
- prevention
- treatment and retention and establishing rapport
- consultation (coordinating with & supporting unit and command
- clinical operations (medical record)

Range of Applications

- types of patients
- policies and procedures
- setting and infrastructure
- garrison/downrange
- various theaters of war (OIF/OEF)

Potential Policymaker Topics

- maintaining situational awareness
- weighing policy actions
- readiness versus health tensions
- interacting with senior DoD and congressional officials

Hindsight and Lessons Learned

- How do you judge the policy and practice changes you described in hindsight?
- What would you do differently if you knew then what you know now?
- If you had to describe specific lessons in terms of preparing to adapt to behavioral health demands in future conflicts, what would they be?

Interview Release Form

The release authorization for our videotaped interviews appears on the next page.

Broad Video Release Authorization for Military Behavioral Health **Lessons Learned**

What am I being asked to Authorize?

RAND would like to record the video and/or phone conversation in which you will be participating and use the recordings for the following purposes:
- Education of external audiences
- Transfer to client (Center for Deployment Psychology), which may place clips of the interview on its website for further education of external audiences

How will the recording be used by RAND?

The audio and video recording will be used solely for the purposes identified in this document. RAND will not use the recordings for any other purpose without your approval. RAND may distribute the recordings in any manner, including by making them available on the internet. You will be identified by name along with the video and/or audio recording. RAND may use the recordings for as long as it would like.

Release Authorization

By signing below, I authorize The RAND Corporation ("RAND") to use video recordings and audio recordings of me to create educational materials about lessons learned in the delivery of military mental health care.

Additionally, I understand and agree that:

- I will be interviewed about my military behavioral health experiences during OIF, OEF, and OND.
- I will be identified by name in conjunction with any video recording or audio recording.
- I will not receive any payment for my appearance in, or RAND's use of, any video recording, or audio recording.
- I am waiving any and all commercial and publicity rights that I may have (or my family or heirs may have) with respect to the video or audio recordings.
- There are no limitations on how the video or audio recordings will be used except as stated in this document.

I am 18 years of age or older and, to the best of my knowledge, am legally capable of entering into agreements in my own name.

Signature: _____ Date: _____

Printed Name: _____

Biographies of the Interviewees

Peter Chiarelli

Peter Chiarelli (General, U.S. Army, retired) was commander of the Multi-National Corps–Iraq, where he coordinated the actions of all four military services and was responsible for the day-to-day combat operations of more than 147,000 U.S. and coalition troops. While serving as the 32nd Vice Chief of Staff in the Army (2008–2012), he was responsible for the day-to-day operations of the Army and its 1.1 million active and reserve soldiers. During this time, he also led DoD efforts on PTSD, TBI, and suicide prevention.

His first assignments were with the 9th Infantry Division at Fort Lewis, including: support platoon leader for 3rd Squadron (Air), 5th Cavalry Regiment; squadron assistant intelligence staff officer (S-2); squadron intelligence staff officer (S-2); troop executive officer; and troop commander.

Chiarelli's principal staff assignments were Operations Officer (G-3), 1st Cavalry Division, at Fort Hood, Texas; Executive Assistant and, later, Executive Officer to the Supreme Allied Commander, Commander U.S. European Command at SHAPE Headquarters, Mons, Belgium; and the Director of Operations, Readiness, and Mobilization (G-3/5/7) at Headquarters, Department of the Army. He commanded a motorized infantry battalion (2nd Battalion, 1st Infantry Regiment) and a motorized infantry brigade (199th Separate Infantry Brigade) at Fort Lewis, Washington; served as the assistant division commander for support in the 1st Cavalry Division at Fort Hood, Texas; served as commanding general, 1st Cavalry Division, and led it both in the Iraq War and during OIF II; and served as commanding general of Multi-National Corps–Iraq.

He holds a B.S. in political science from Seattle University, an M.P.A. from the Daniel J. Evans School of Public Affairs at the University of Washington, and an M.A. in national security strategy from Salve Regina University. He is also a graduate of the U.S. Naval Command and Staff College and the National War College.

In 2018, he retired as chief executive officer of One Mind, which is dedicated to benefiting all affected by brain illness and injury through fostering fundamental changes.

David Chu

David S. C. Chu, Ph.D., served as president of the Institute for Defense Analyses from 2009 to 2019, where he continues as an adjunct staff member. In DoD, he served as Under Secretary of Defense for Personnel and Readiness (2001–2009) and, earlier, as Assistant Secretary of Defense and Director for Program Analysis and Evaluation (1981–1993). From 1978 to 1981, he was the assistant director of the Congressional Budget Office for National Security and International Affairs. He began his career as a U.S. Army officer (1968–1970). He was an economist with the RAND Corporation (1970–1978), director of its Washington Office (1994–1998), and vice president for its Army Research Division (1998–2001). He earned his Ph.D. in economics from Yale University. He is a member of the Defense Science Board and a fellow of the National Academy of Public Administration. He is a recipient of the DoD Medal for Distinguished Public Service with Gold Palm, the Department of Veterans Affairs Meritorious Service Award, the Department of the Army Distinguished Civilian Service Award, the Department of the Navy Distinguished Public Service Award, and the National Academy of Public Administration's National Public Service Award.

Bruce Crow

Bruce Crow, Psy.D., M.P.H. (colonel, U.S. Army, retired), is a clinical psychologist with a long-standing career focus on military and veteran behavioral health. He currently serves as the associate director of program evaluation for the Department of Veterans Affairs Suicide Prevention Program and recently completed a research fellowship in dissemination and implementation science at the University of Washington School of Medicine. He holds a Psy.D. from Nova Southeastern University and a Master of Public Health from the University of North Texas Health Sciences Center.

Crow served with the U.S. Army for 30 years, retiring from active duty in 2012 at the rank of colonel. He continued with the Army as a civilian psychologist for five years, leading development of DoD's largest tele-behavioral health operation. While on active duty, he completed a post-doctoral fellowship in clinical neuropsychology and held several senior leadership positions within the military, including eight years as the Army's chief psychologist. He has served as a military subject-matter expert in posttraumatic stress, deployment psychology, suicide prevention, and tele–behavioral health, with specific expertise in designing and implementing suicide reduction initiatives for behavioral health providers. Crow has served as a subject-matter expert consultant for military psychology and military suicide to the ministries of defense for Australia, Estonia, and Columbia. He currently serves on the Executive Committee of APA's Division of Military Psychology and serves as chair of the Public Health Committee of the American Association of Suicidology. He is a 2018 recipient of the John C. Flanagan Lifetime Achievement Award from APA Division 19 (Society for Military Psychology).

Michael Dinneen

Michael Dinneen, M.D., Ph.D., has been director of the Office of Strategy Management for the MHS since he retired from the U.S. Navy in January 2005. Following his medical training, he was a staff psychiatrist. He then transferred to the NNMC, where he was first a director of residency training, then chairman of the Department of Psychiatry, and finally director of medical services. When Congress threatened to outsource all military mental health care in the National Capital Area, he developed and implemented a strategic plan to reduce psychiatric hospital beds from 200 to 60 while actually increasing the military's share of the mental health market. Subsequent changes resulted in an integrated training and service-delivery program that provided expanded child and adolescent services. At the same time, overall operating expenses were reduced by more than 30 percent. Dinneen was also a special psychiatric consultant to the Secret Service and U.S. State Department, the attending physician to Congress, National Organization for Victim Assistance, and Office of the White House Physician. He developed his special expertise in psychological trauma and military psychiatry while leading Navy Special Psychiatric Rapid Intervention Teams for more than 10 years, directing Mental Health Services aboard the hospital ship USNS *Comfort* during Desert Shield/Desert Storm, and treating service members and their families. He has lectured internationally on traumatic stress, developed curricula in trauma psychiatry, and trained personnel for specialized wartime assignments. His publications on psychological trauma include original research on the effects of exposure to the stresses of deployment during Desert Shield and Desert Storm. In 2002, Dinneen became director of health care planning and TRICARE operations at the Navy Bureau of Medicine. He implemented a standard business planning process for the Navy's 38 medical treatment facilities and was responsible for the orderly transition to the new generation of TRICARE contracts. A diplomate of the American Board of Psychiatry and Neurology, Dinneen graduated from Harvard University (*cum laude*) and received both an M.D. and Ph.D. (in neurochemistry) from the Medical College of Virginia.[1]

---

[1]   Adapted from Appendix A of Butler et al., 2009.

Charles Engel

Charles Engel, M.D., M.P.H. (colonel, U.S. Army, retired), is a senior physician policy researcher at RAND. As a psychiatrist and health services researcher, his work focuses on trauma-informed health systems and strategies for improving quality of care for chronic mental and physical health conditions. His research in general medical settings, including primary care, has covered traumatic injury and trauma syndromes and symptoms, including blast injury, polytrauma, mild TBI, postconcussive syndrome, Gulf War syndrome, PTSD and depression. Engel uses mixed qualitative and quantitative research methods relating to pragmatic randomized trials, knowledge readiness and research impact assessment, program evaluation, and implementation science. He has authored or coauthored more than 180 scholarly articles, including in the *New England Journal of Medicine*, the *Journal of the American Medical Association*, and the *American Journal of Psychiatry*. Funding for Engel's research has come from the National Institutes of Health, Centers for Disease Control, the VA, DoD, and other agencies. Before RAND, Engel was associate chair for research for the Uniformed Services University Department of Psychiatry. Engel has served on the Board of Directors of the International Society for Traumatic Stress Studies, has delivered more than 200 invited presentations in 11 countries, and is a recipient of the Porter Award from the Association of Military Surgeons of the United States for contributions to psychiatry in the military. Engel received his M.P.H. from the University of Washington School of Public Health and his M.D. from the University of Washington School of Medicine.

Eric Getka

Eric J. Getka, Ph.D. (captain, Medical Service Corps, U.S. Navy, retired), earned his B.S. (Summa Cum Laude) in Psychology from Loyola University of Maryland in 1978. He earned his M.A. and Ph.D. in Clinical Psychology from the Catholic University of America. Early in his doctoral studies, he was selected for acceptance into the Navy's Health Professions Scholarship Program.

Getka's first assignment on active duty was at the NNMC for his doctoral internship (October 1981–October 1982). Following his internship, Getka transferred to the Navy Medical Clinic, Quantico, Virginia, where he served as staff psychologist (October 1982–January 1984). His next assignment was as head of Behavioral Health Care at the Navy Postgraduate Dental Center, Bethesda, Maryland, from January 1984 to July 1986. In July 1986, he was assigned as Outpatient Department head, Tri-Service Alcohol Rehabilitation Program at the NNMC. After assignment to the Naval Hospital, Yokosuka, Japan, in November 1988, he headed the Substance Abuse Rehabilitation Department.

Following his assignment in Japan, he was selected for a two-year postdoctoral fellowship in clinical neuropsychology at the Georgetown University Medical Center in Washington, D.C. After completing his fellowship in December 1993, he transferred back to the NNMC, where he served as head of Neuropsychological Services. During that tour, Getka also commenced a three-year appointment as Specialty Advisor to the Navy Surgeon General for Clinical Psychology (1999–2003).

In 2001, he moved to the Navy Medical Center, San Diego, California, where he headed the Substance Abuse Rehabilitation Department and, later, headed Mental Health Services. He retired from active duty in 2005 and was selected as the national director for Navy Psychology Training and Recruitment Programs. He retired from federal service in March 2019.

His military awards and decorations include the Meritorious Service Medal, Navy Commendation Medal (two awards), Navy Achievement Medal, Meritorious Unit Commendation, National Defense Service Medal, Global War on Terrorism Service Medal, and the Navy/Marine Corps Overseas Service Ribbon.

Carroll Greene

Carroll Greene III, Ph.D. (colonel U.S. Air Force, retired), is a member of the American Board of Professional Psychology and an award-winning executive with over 40 years of behavioral health and operational military experience. He has served for more than nine years at the U.S. Marine Raider Training Center and is the director of psychological applications. He developed and leads psychological applications to enhance individual and unit performance in the assessment, selection, and training of Marine special operations personnel. His 24-plus years of military and civilian service in U.S. Special Operations Command has included clinical health care leadership and operational support to combat and intelligence operations. He has developed and managed applications for special-access programs and top-tier special mission forces and acted as a consultant to commanders on unique operational and personnel performance challenges for both air and ground forces, in garrison and deployed. As the first psychologist assigned to newly formed Air Force Special Operations Command in 1993 and, later, the first psychologist assigned to several special mission units within the Joint Special Operations Command 1998 through 2004, he helped shape the historical growth of behavioral health and operational psychology applications for U.S. Special Operations Command.

David Kieran

David Kieran, Ph.D., is an assistant professor of history and director of the American Studies Concentration at Washington and Jefferson College in Washington, Pennsylvania. He studies war and society in U.S. culture, with a particular interest in the legacies of the Vietnam War and the United States' 21st-century wars. He is the author, most recently, of *Signature Wounds: The Untold Story of the Military's Mental Health Crisis* (New York University Press, 2019), the research and writing for which was supported by the National Endowment for the Humanities and a Tanner Fellowship at the University of Utah. His first book was *Forever Vietnam: How a Divisive War Changed Ameri-*

can Public Memory (University of Massachusetts Press, 2014). He is also the editor of *The War of My Generation: Youth Culture and the War on Terror* (Rutgers University Press, 2015), and he is the coeditor, with Edwin A. Martini, of *At War: The Military and American Culture in the Twentieth Century and Beyond* (Rutgers University Press, 2018) and, with Rebecca A. Adelman, of a special issue of *The Journal of War and Culture Studies* on the topic "New Cultures of Remote Warfare" and *Remote Warfare: New Cultures of Violence* (University of Minnesota Press, 2020). He is currently working on two projects: a history of the National Guard in the 21st century wars and a book manuscript tentatively entitled *Let All the Wounds of War Be Healed: The Amnesty Debate and the Aftermath of the Vietnam War*. He earned his B.A. at Connecticut College and his Ph.D. in American Studies at The George Washington University.

Robert Lippy

Robert D. Lippy, Ph.D. (commander, Medical Service Corps, U.S. Navy), is a member of the American Board of Professional Psychology. He enlisted in the Navy in 1989 as an electronics technician. After serving for almost four years and attaining the rank of E-5, he received a Navy ROTC scholarship to attend Oregon State University, graduating in 1996 with a B.S. in psychology and receiving his commission as a surface warfare officer. After completing Division officer training at surface Warfare Officer School in Newport, Rhode Island, he was stationed in San Diego for almost six years, serving aboard various amphibious warfare ships and making several Western Pacific and Indian Ocean deployments. During this period, he earned his Surface Warfare Officer qualification, served as a naval beach group officer in command and became a Navy master training specialist, teaching an expeditionary warfare staff planning course to operational sailors and marines.

He was then selected to attend graduate training at USUHS in Bethesda, Maryland, where he received his M.S. and his Ph.D. in clinical psychology in 2005 and 2008, respectively. He completed his clinical internship and a year of postdoctoral training at the NNMC.

From 2008 to 2011 he was stationed at Naval Medical Center San Diego, serving as a staff psychologist at two branch mental health clinics and as the division officer of the Adult Outpatient Mental Health Clinic. In 2010, he deployed to Afghanistan as an individual augmentee with 1st Medical Battalion from Camp Pendleton, California. He served as the officer in charge of the Combat Stress Clinic at Camp Dwyer, Helmand Province, where he helped establish its Warrior Recovery Center while earning his Fleet Marine Force Officer qualification.

He transferred to the USS *Carl Vinson* aircraft carrier (CVN 70) in 2011, where he completed a six-month Western Pacific and Indian Ocean deployment and earned his Surface Warfare Medical Department Officer qualification. From 2013 to 2017 he was stationed at Naval Hospital Camp Pendleton, California, where he headed the Mental Health Department and was selected as the Officer of the Year for 2015. That same year, he was selected by the clinical psychology specialty leader to be the subspecialty leader for embedded navy psychologists (serving on aircraft carriers and with submarine squadrons).

Lippy is currently the deputy director of the Naval Center for Combat and Operational Stress Control, whose mission is to optimize the psychological readiness of sailors and marines through the development, aggregation, and dissemination of best practices and innovations in primary, secondary, and tertiary prevention of psychological injury and disease. In 2018, he was also selected to chair the Navy Psychological Health Clinical Community, leading the entire psychological health community of over 700 active-duty providers and behavioral health technicians, as well as thousands of civilian mental health professionals across Navy Medicine, in implementation of leading practices, informing policy, and supporting the psychological health community in securing Navy Medicine's readiness mission by delivering the highest quality of care to all beneficiaries. In recognition of his accomplishments, Lippy was selected as the 2018 Navy Senior Psychologist of the Year, as well as the 2019 Military Health System Allied Health Leadership Excellence Award (Senior Provider).

Lippy is board certified in clinical psychology. Among his military awards are the Meritorious Service Medal, Navy Commendation Medal (three awards), Navy Achievement Medal (four awards), and the Global War on Terrorism Medal.

William Nash

William P. Nash, M.D., is a clinical and research psychiatrist at the VA Greater Los Angeles Healthcare System, and a Health Sciences Associate Clinical Professor at the David Geffen School of Medicine at the University of California at Los Angeles, where he leads an emerging program of research and treatment for veterans with moral injury. Previously, he served as the director of psychological health for the U.S. Marine Corps and, while on active duty in the Navy, as combat-stress-control psychiatrist embedded with the 1st Marine Division in Iraq. The doctrine for maintaining psychological health in military operations that Nash wrote in 2008 still informs leadership training throughout the U.S. Navy and Marine Corps. His peer-reviewed research with Marine infantrymen was the first to document PTSD in service members as a direct result of violations of moral expectations. He has coauthored two books, *Combat Stress Injury: Theory, Research, and Management* (2007), and *Adaptive Disclosure: A New Treatment for Military Trauma, Loss, and Moral Injury* (2017).

David Orman

David Orman, M.D. (colonel, U.S. Army, retired), is currently a DHA civil-service employee serving as the clinical director of the Behavioral Health System of Care at Joint Base San Antonio–Fort Sam Houston, Texas. His role within DHA's behavioral health clinical management team is to provide strategic planning for DHA's evolving Behavioral

Health System of Care and to provide operational program management for the DHA's behavioral health prevention and clinical services.

He brings the depth of about 38 years active duty Army and civilian administrative, academic, educational, and research experience to his current position. Prior roles include serving for eight years as the Army Surgeon General's psychiatry consultant, program director for Psychiatric Graduate Medical Education at Tripler Army Medical Center in Honolulu-Oahu, Hawaii, and associate program director and associate professor for Texas A&M School of Medicine/Scott & White's psychiatry residency. He has also served as chief of psychiatry at Brooke Army Medical Center–San Antonio and Darnall Army Community Hospital–Fort Hood, Texas, and as the division psychiatrist for the 1st Cavalry Division. He retired as a colonel after 30 years of service in 2007 and has been in his current civil service position in various roles since October 2007. Just prior to his military retirement in 2007, he worked for approximately one year as part of the DoD Task Force that ultimately resulted in Congress supplementing DoD's behavioral health–TBI clinical services budgets in all three services by approximately $900 million.

Orman received his medical school education thorough USUHS in Bethesda, Maryland, and completed his four-year psychiatry residency training at Walter Reed Army Medical Center, Washington, D.C., where he served as chief resident in 1985. He is the coauthor of numerous publications.

Mark Paris

Mark Paris, Ph.D, earned his doctorate at Louisiana State University and had a clinical postdoctoral fellowship at the University of Southern Mississippi. He then became an Army officer and completed a clinical internship at Dwight David Eisenhower Army Medical at Fort Gordon, Georgia. Following seven additional years as an Army clinical psychologist, he worked for the next 20 years as a mental health policy analyst in the Office of the Assistant Secretary of Defense (Health Affairs) before completing his federal service as the Director of Psychological Health for the Army's Regional Health Command–Atlantic. Paris is currently in a part-time consulting practice, serving both the VA and the Social Security Administration. He holds the Diplomate in Clinical Psychology from the American Board of Professional Psychology and is licensed in both Maryland and Virginia.

Rebecca Porter

Rebecca I. Porter, Ph.D. (colonel, U.S. Army, retired), has been the president and chief executive officer of the Military Child Education Coalition since September 2019.

Her initial Army tour was as a clerk typist in the Washington Army National Guard in Seattle, Washington, from 1981 to 1983. Her first assignment on active duty was in 1984 as a platoon leader in the 272d Military Police Company in Kaefertal, Germany. From 1985 to 1987, she served as the adjutant and personnel officer of the 95th Military Police Battalion in Mannheim, Germany, before entering the U.S. Army Reserve as an assistant Operations Officer and Detachment Commander in the 448th Civil Affairs Battalion at Fort Lewis, Washington.

In June 1995, she returned to active duty as a clinical psychology intern at Tripler Army Medical Center in Honolulu, Hawaii. Following the completion of her doctorate in clinical psychology, she stayed at Tripler as the chief of the Chronic Pain Program. From 1997 to 1999, she served at Fort Bliss, Texas, as the chief of community mental health. In 1999, she transferred to the Pentagon, where she served first as an operations officer and liaison officer in the Office of the Chief of Legislative Liaison and, from 2001 to 2003, as a special assistant to GEN Eric K. Shinseki, then serving as the Army's 34th Chief of Staff.

From 2003 to 2005, she completed a postdoctoral fellowship in clinical health psychology and then served as the director of Psychology Fellowship Programs. From 2005 to 2007, she was director of the Center for Personal Development at the U.S. Military Academy at West Point, New York. In 2007 and 2008, she was deployed with Joint Task Force 34 in Iraq. On her redeployment, Porter served as the chief of psychology at Walter Reed Army Medical Center in Washington, D.C. From 2009 to 2010, she was the staff behavioral health officer of Joint Task Force Capital Medical. Following that assignment, Porter transferred to the OTSG from 2010 to 2013.

From 2013 to 2015, she commanded Dunham U.S. Army Health Clinic, with facilities in four Pennsylvania locations: Carlisle Barracks, Fort Indiantown Gap, Letterkenny Army Depot, and New Cumberland. Following that command, she was the director of the DiLorenzo TRICARE Health Clinic of the Pentagon from 2015 to 2016. She commanded the Public Health Command Europe from July 2017 to July 2019.

She is a 1983 Distinguished Military Graduate from the University of Washington. She holds an M.A. in counseling psychology from Chapman University, a Ph.D. in clinical psychology from Fielding Graduate University, and an M.S. in national security and strategic studies from the National War College. With more than three decades of military service, She is a board-certified clinical health psychologist, a fellow of the American Psychological Association, and a member of the Order of Military Medical Merit. Her awards include the Lifetime Achievement Award from the Society for Military Psychology, the Legion of Merit (three awards), the Defense Meritorious Service Medal, and the Meritorious Service Medal (six awards). She also holds the Surgeon General's "A" proficiency designator as recognition of her significant contributions to the Army Medical Department.

David Riggs

David Riggs, Ph.D., is professor and chair, Department of Medical and Clinical Psychology at the F. Edward Hérbert School of Medicine at the USUHS, where he is also executive director of the CDP. As professor and chair, he leads a program to train active-duty and civilian psychology students to deliver outstanding patient care and contribute to clinically relevant science in psychology. As executive director of the CDP, he oversees the development and delivery of training seminars and workshops for behavioral health professionals to prepare them to provide for the needs of warriors and their families. Previously, he held clinical research positions at the Center for the Treatment and Study of Anxiety at the University of Pennsylvania and the National Center for Posttraumatic Stress Disorder at the Boston Veterans Administration Medical Center. As a clinical and research psychologist, much of his work has focused on trauma, violence, and anxiety, with a particular interest in the effects of PTSD and other anxiety disorders on the families of those directly affected.

Eric Schoomaker

Eric Schoomaker, M.D., Ph.D. (lieutenant general, U.S. Army retired), is the director of the USUHS Leadership Education and Development program. After four years as the U.S. Army's top medical officer, he retired in 2012 from his role as the 42nd U.S. Army Surgeon General and commanding general of MEDCOM. This followed 32 years of active service in uniform and 41 years as a commissioned Army officer. He is exploring the central importance of leadership education and training for health professionals in both individual career development for different health professions—uniformed and civilian—and in an interprofessional, team-based setting.

He was sworn in as Army Surgeon General after commanding Walter Reed Army Medical Center and North Atlantic Regional Medical Command in Washington, D.C. He received a B.S. from the University of Michigan in 1970 and was commissioned as a second lieutenant as a Distinguished Military Graduate. He received his medical degree from the University of Michigan in 1975 and a Ph.D. in human genetics in 1979. He completed an internal medicine internship and residency at Duke University Medical Center in North Carolina from 1976–1978, followed by a fellowship in hematology at Duke in 1979. He is certified by the American Board of Internal Medicine in both internal medicine and hematology.

While in uniform, he held many assignments, including chief and program director, Department of Medicine and director of Primary Care, Madigan Army Medical Center, Fort Lewis, Washington;

commander of the Evans Army Community Hospital at Fort Carson, Colorado; commander, 30th Medical Brigade and Fifth Corps Surgeon in Heidelberg, Germany; chief of the Army Medical Corps; commander of the Southeast Regional Medical Command/Dwight David Eisenhower Army Medical Center in Fort Gordon, Georgia; and commanding general of the U.S. Army Medical Research & Materiel Command & Fort Detrick, Maryland. He is the recipient of numerous military awards, including those from France and Germany, the 2012 Dr. Nathan Davis Awards from the American Medical Association for outstanding government service, the Philipp M. Lippe, MD Award from the American Academy of Pain Medicine for contributions to the social and political aspect of pain medicine, and an Honorary Doctor of Science from Wake Forest University.

Terri Tanielian

Terri Tanielian is a senior behavioral scientist and an internationally recognized expert on military and veterans' health policy. Her areas of interest include military and veterans' health policy; military suicide; military sexual assault; and the psychological effects of combat, terrorism, and disasters. She has led multiple studies to assess the needs of veterans and to examine the readiness of private health care providers to deliver timely, high quality care to veterans and their families. She has also examined community-based models for expanding mental health care for returning veterans and their families.

As the former director of the RAND Center for Military Health Policy Research, she spent a decade overseeing RAND's diverse military health research portfolio. She was the co–study director for a large, nongovernmental assessment of the psychological, emotional, and cognitive consequences of deployment to Iraq and Afghanistan entitled *Invisible Wounds of War: Psychological and Cognitive Injuries, Their Consequences, and Services to Assist Recovery* (RAND, 2008). She was also the codirector for the RAND study that produced *Hidden Heroes: America's Military Caregivers* (Ramchand, Tanielian, et al., 2014), the first representative examination of military caregiving in the United

States. She also recently completed a feasibility assessment examining the integration of DoD and VA purchased care approaches.

Tanielian has published numerous peer-reviewed articles and reports. She currently serves as a fellow in the Military Service Initiative for the George W. Bush Institute. She was a member of the planning committee for the 18th, 22nd, and 26th Annual Rosalynn Carter Symposiums on Mental Health Policy, which focused on mental health needs and recovery following 9/11, Hurricane Katrina, and deployment to Iraq and Afghanistan, respectively. She earned her M.A. in psychology at American University.

Jonathan Woodson

Jonathan Woodson, M.D. (brigadier general, U.S. Army Reserve), was the Assistant Secretary of Defense for Health Affairs. In this role, he administered the more than $50 billion MHS budget and served as principal advisor to the Secretary of Defense for health issues. The MHS comprises over 133,000 military and civilian doctors, nurses, medical educators, researchers, healthcare providers, allied health professionals, and health administration personnel worldwide, providing our nation with an unequalled integrated healthcare delivery, expeditionary medical, educational, and research capability.

He ensured the effective execution of the DoD medical mission. He oversaw the development of medical policies, analyses, and recommendations to the Secretary of Defense and the Undersecretary for Personnel and Readiness and issued guidance to DoD components on medical matters. He also served as the principal advisor to the Undersecretary for Personnel and Readiness on matters of chemical, biological, radiological, and nuclear medical defense programs and deployment matters pertaining to force health.

He cochairs the Armed Services Biomedical Research Evaluation and Management Committee, which facilitates oversight of DoD biomedical research. In addition, he exercises authority, direction, and control over DHA; USUHS; the Armed Forces Radiobiology Research

Institute; DCoE; the Armed Forces Institute of Pathology; and the Armed Services Blood Program Office.

Prior to his appointment by President Barack Obama, he was associate dean for Diversity and Multicultural Affairs and professor of surgery at the Boston University School of Medicine and senior attending vascular surgeon at Boston Medical Center. He has served as Assistant Surgeon General for Reserve Affairs, Force Structure and Mobilization in the OTSG, and as Deputy Commander of the Army Reserve Medical Command.

He is a graduate of the City College of New York and the New York University School of Medicine. He received his postgraduate medical education at the Massachusetts General Hospital, Harvard Medical School and completed residency training in internal medicine and general and vascular surgery. He is board certified in internal medicine, general surgery, vascular surgery, and critical care surgery. He also holds an M.S.S. in strategic studies (concentration in strategic leadership) from the U.S. Army War College.

In 1992, he was awarded a research fellowship at the Association of American Medical Colleges Health Services Research Institute. He has authored or coauthored a number of publications and book chapters on vascular trauma and outcomes in vascular limb salvage surgery.

His prior military assignments include deployments to Saudi Arabia (Operation Desert Storm), Kosovo, OEF, and OIF. He has also served as a senior medical officer with the National Disaster Management System, where he responded to the 9/11 attack in New York City. Woodson's military awards and decorations include the Legion of Merit, the Bronze Star Medal, and the Meritorious Service Medal (with oak leaf cluster).

In 2007, he was named one of the top vascular surgeons in Boston and, in 2008, was listed as one of the top surgeons in the U.S. He is the recipient of the 2009 Gold Humanism in Medicine Award from the Association of American Medical Colleges.

Abbreviations

APA	American Psychological Association
BHDP	Behavioral Health Data Portal
BSC	behavioral science consultant
BSCT	behavioral science consultant team
CDP	Center for Deployment Psychology
CSC	combat stress control
DCoE	Defense Centers of Excellence for Psychological Health and Traumatic Brain Injury
DHA	Defense Health Agency
DoD	U.S. Department of Defense
DoDI	DoD Instruction
FY	fiscal year
MEDCOM	Army Medical Command
MHAT	mental health advisory team
MHS	Military Health System
MTF	military treatment facility
NDAA	National Defense Authorization Act

NNMC	National Naval Medical Center
OEF	Operation Enduring Freedom
OIF	Operation Iraqi Freedom
OPTEMPO	operational tempo
OTSG	Office of the Surgeon General
PTSD	posttraumatic stress disorder
TBI	traumatic brain injury
USUHS	Uniformed Services University of the Health Sciences
VA	Department of Veterans Affairs

References

Adler, Amy B., Paul D. Bliese, Dennis McGurk, Charles W. Hoge, and Carl Andrew Castro, "Battlemind Debriefing and Battlemind Training as Early Interventions with Soldiers Returning from Iraq: Randomization by Platoon," *Journal of Consulting and Clinical Psychology*, Vol. 77, No. 5, 2009, pp. 928–940. As of July 16, 2020:
https://doi.org/10.1037/a0016877

American Psychological Association, "Timeline of APA Policies & Actions Related to Detainee Welfare and Professional Ethics in the Context of Interrogation and National Security," webpage, undated. As of July 16, 2020:
https://www.apa.org/news/press/statements/interrogations

———, *Report of the American Psychological Association Presidential Task Force on Psychological Ethics and National Security*, Washington, D.C., June 2005. As of July 21, 2020:
https://www.apa.org/pubs/info/reports/pens.pdf

———, "Chapter XIV. International Affairs," webpage, 2008.

APA—*See* American Psychological Association.

Butler, David, Jessica Buono, Frederick Erdtmann, and Proctor Reid, eds., *Systems Engineering to Improve Traumatic Brain Injury Care in the Military Health System: Workshop Summary*, Washington, D.C.: National Academies Press, 2009.

CDP—*See* Center for Deployment Psychology.

Center for Deployment Psychology, "About CDP," webpage, undated. As of November 24, 2020:
https://deploymentpsych.org/about/main

Defense Health Agency Procedural Instruction 6490.02, *Behavioral Health (BH) Treatment and Outcomes Monitoring*, July 12, 2018. As of November 24, 2020:
https://health.mil/Reference-Center/Policies/2018/07/12/
DHA-PI-6490-01-BH-Treatment-and-Outcomes-Monitoring

Department of Defense Directive 3115.09, *DoD Intelligence Interrogations, Detainee Debriefings, and Tactical Questioning*, Washington, D.C.: U.S. Department of Defense, November 3, 2005. As of July 16, 2020:
https://fas.org/irp/doddir/dod/d3115_09-2005.pdf

Department of Defense Form DD Form 2796, "Post-Deployment Health Assessment," April 2003. As of November 23, 2020:
https://www.jiatfs.southcom.mil/Portals/4/Documents/J4/J4_dd2796.pdf

Department of Defense Instruction 2310.08E, *Medical Program Support for Detainee Operations*, Washington, D.C.: U.S. Department of Defense, June 6, 2006. As of July 6, 2006:
http://hrlibrary.umn.edu/OathBetrayed/Winkenwerder%206-6-2006.pdf

Department of Defense Instruction 6490.08, *Command Notification Requirements to Dispel Stigma in Providing Mental Health Care to Service Members*, August 17, 2011. As of July 16, 2020:
https://www.esd.whs.mil/Portals/54/Documents/DD/issuances/dodi/649008p.pdf

Department of Defense Instruction 6490.09, *DoD Directors of Psychological Health*, February 27, 2012 (change 2 dated April 25, 2017). As of November 24, 2020:
https://www.esd.whs.mil/Portals/54/Documents/DD/issuances/dodi/
649009p.pdf?ver=2019-04-03-145810-913

Department of Defense Task Force on Mental Health, *An Achievable Vision*, Falls Church, Va.: Defense Health Board, 2007. As of July 16, 2020:
https://www.pdhealth.mil/strategy-policy-library/
achievable-vision-report-department-defense-task-force-mental-health-june-2007

Directive Type Memorandum 09-033, *Policy Guidance for Management of Concussion/Mild Traumatic Brain Injury in the Deployed Setting*, Washington, D.C.: U.S. Department of Defense, June 21, 2010.

DoDI—*See* Department of Defense Instruction.

Hoffman, David H., Danielle J. Carter, Cara R. Viglucci Lopez, Heather L. Benzmiller, Ava X. Guo, S. Yasir Latifi, and Daniel C. Craig, *Report to the Special Committee of the Board of Directors of the American Psychological Association: Independent Review Relating to APA Ethics Guidelines, National Security Interrogations, and Torture*, Washington, D.C.: Sidley Austin LLP, July 2, 2015. As of July 16, 2020:
https://www.apa.org/independent-review/revised-report.pdf

Hoge, Charles W., Christopher G. Ivany, Edward A. Brusher, Millard D. Brown III, John C. Shero, Amy B. Adler, Christopher H. Warner, and David T. Orman, "Transformation of Mental Health Care for U.S. Soldiers and Families During the Iraq and Afghanistan Wars: Where Science and Politics Intersect," *American Journal of Psychiatry*, Vol. 173, No. 4, April 2016, pp. 334–343. As of July 16, 2020:
https://ajp.psychiatryonline.org/doi/full/10.1176/appi.ajp.2015.15040553

Kieran, David, *Signature Wounds: The Untold Story of the Military's Mental Health Crisis*, New York: New York University Press, 2019.

Management of Post-Traumatic Stress Working Group, *VA/DoD Clinical Practice Guideline for the Management of Post-Traumatic Stress*, Vers. 1.0, Washington, D.C.: Department of Veterans Affairs and Department of Defense, January 2004. As of November 24, 2020:
https://www.healthquality.va.gov/ptsd/ptsd_full.pdf

OIF MHAT—*See* Operation Iraqi Freedom Mental Health Advisory Team.

Office of the Surgeon General, *Behavioral Science Consultation Policy*, Fort Sam Houston, Tex.: Headquarters, U.S. Army Medical Command, Policy Memo 06-029, October 20, 2006. As of November 24, 2020:
http://www.ethicalpsychology.org/materials/
otsg_medcom_policy_06-029-bsct_2006.pdf

————, *Behavioral Science Consultation Policy*, Fort Sam Houston, Tex., Headquarters, U.S. Army Medical Command, OTSG/MEDCOM policy memo 09–053, 2009.

————, *Behavioral Science Consultation Policy*, Falls Church, Va.: U.S. Department of the Army, OTSG/MEDCOM policy memo 13–027, 2013.

Operation Iraqi Freedom Mental Health Advisory Team, *Operation Iraqi Freedom (OIF) Mental Health Advisory Team (MHAT) Report*, U.S. Army Surgeon General & HQDA G-1, December 16, 2003. As of July 16, 2020:
https://www-tc.pbs.org/wgbh/pages/frontline/shows/heart/readings/mhat.pdf

OTSG—*See* Office of the Surgeon General.

President's Commission on Care for America's Returning Wounded Warriors, *Serve, Support, Simplify*, Washington, D.C., 2007.

Public Law 109-364, John Warner National Defense Authorization Act for Fiscal Year 2007, October 17, 2006. As of July 21, 2020:
https://www.congress.gov/109/plaws/publ364/PLAW-109publ364.pdf

Public Law 110-417, Duncan Hunter National Defense Authorization Act for Fiscal Year 2009, October 14, 2008. As of July 16, 2020:
https://www.congress.gov/110/plaws/publ417/PLAW-110publ417.pdf

Public Law 111-84, National Defense Authorization Act for Fiscal Year 2010, October 28, 2009. As of November 24, 2020:
https://www.govinfo.gov/content/pkg/PLAW-111publ84/pdf/
PLAW-111publ84.pdf

Public Law 112-81, National Defense Authorization Act for Fiscal Year 2012, December 31, 2011. As of July 21, 2020:
https://www.congress.gov/112/plaws/publ81/PLAW-112publ81.pdf

Ramchand, Rajeev, Terri Tanielian, Michael P. Fisher, Christine Anne Vaughan, Thomas E. Trail, Caroline Epley, Phoenix Voorhies, Michael William Robbins, Eric Robinson, Bonnie Ghosh-Dastidar, *Hidden Heroes: America's Military Caregivers*, Santa Monica, Calif.: RAND Corporation, RR-499-TEDF, 2014. As of November 24, 2020:
https://www.rand.org/pubs/research_reports/RR499.html

Reger, Greg M., and Bret A. Moore, "Combat Operational Stress Control in Iraq: Lessons Learned During Operation Iraqi Freedom," *Military Psychology*, Vol. 18, No. 4, 2006, pp. 297–307. As of December 4, 2020:
https://www.tandfonline.com/doi/full/10.1207/s15327876mp1804_4

Tanielian, Terri and Lisa H. Jaycox, eds., *Invisible Wounds of War: Psychological and Cognitive Injuries, Their Consequences, and Services to Assist Recovery*, Santa Monica, Calif.: RAND Corporation, MG-720-CCF, 2008. As of November 21, 2020:
https://www.rand.org/pubs/monographs/MG720.html

U.S. Army Center for Health Promotion and Preventive Medicine, *Investigation of Homicides at Fort Carson, Colorado November 2008–May 2009*, Aberdeen Proving Ground, Md., Epidemiologic Consultation No. 14-HK-OB1U-09, July 2009. As of July 16, 2020:
https://apps.dtic.mil/sti/pdfs/ADA515975.pdf

U.S. Government Accountability Office, Defense Health: Coordinating Authority Needed for Psychological Health and Traumatic Brain Injury Activities, Washington, D.C., GAO-12-154, January 2012. As of November 23, 2020:
https://www.gao.gov/assets/590/587919.pdf

Williams, Thomas J., and W. Brad Johnson, "Introduction to the Special Issue: Operational Psychology and Clinical Practice in Operational Environments," *Military Psychology*, Vol. 18, No. 4, 2006, pp. 261–268. As of December 4, 2020:
https://www.tandfonline.com/doi/full/10.1207/s15327876mp1804_1